MW01101372

To Sue (handwritten)

THE F.I.T. FILES
Balance it out

SUE COMEAU

THE F.I.T. FILES
BALANCE IT OUT

Copyright © 2014 by Sue Comeau

Printed in Canada.

Cover Design and Interior Format

For Tom and CC.
Love you like crazy.

CHAPTER 1

I was standing in center court at Wimbledon. The stands were packed. I shook my opponents hand, then raised my arms and smiled as the crowd went crazy.

It had taken me five sets, but I was the youngest Wimbledon champion ever. It still hadn't sunk in.

For some reason, the high school girls' tennis team was there. The captain, Carolina, handed me my golden winner's plate. She was wearing her varsity tennis team uniform and her golden blond hair was pulled back in a ponytail.

I looked over and saw The Black Eyed Peas. Bruno Mars and Taylor Swift were there too. They were all giving me thumbs up signs and then they started singing. Everyone started chanting my name...

"Finn! Finn! Finn!"

Carolina smiled and said my name as she leaned in to kiss me on the cheek...

"You rock Finn..."

Finn.

"Finn!"

"Finn! I'm getting the ice cubes if I don't hear your feet on the floor!"

I opened one eye halfway. It was the sound of my dad's *way* too cheerful voice from downstairs.

Man, my favorite dream interrupted again!

The morning ice cube approach is very simple yet effective: a handful of ice cubes under the covers. Not fun. My grandfather used to do it to Dad when he was thirteen - my age – and wouldn't haul his butt out of bed.

Luckily, Gramps also told me one of Dad's tricks. So I followed suit and put one of my feet on the floor while the rest of me was still cozy in bed, and stamped it on the ground. Oh man, way too much energy expenditure for being half asleep.

"I'm up!" I yelled. I stamped my foot a few more times for authenticity. All Dad needed to hear was feet on the ground, and he left me alone. I can't believe he falls for his own trick, but that's the way the ball bounces.

What time was it, five a.m. or something? I looked over the big lug of a dog that was snuggled beside me, at my clock. Ugh, 7:25.

I settled in for a few minutes of shut-eye, trying to nudge Ralph, my Labrador retriever over, when I heard the 'ting' of my cell phone. If Dad only knew: Nothing gets me up quicker than a text.

I got up and picked up my phone. It was from my best friend, Charlie.

NEED 2 C U!! PICK U UP 4 SKUL.

Considering he picks me up for school every

morning, it must be something important, probably related to his 'emergency' (he has a flare for drama) phone call last night.

I put down my phone and looked in the mirror, bleary-eyed. I ran my fingers through my hair. Hmm, I needed a haircut. I stretched and yawned. I had been playing some extra tennis lately, my favorite sport. I wondered if my racket arm was getting bigger.

"AH-NYAH-HA-HA-HAAAA!"

Fiona, my darling sister (yes, I'm being facetious), burst into my room, looked at me, and started laughing like a maniac as she ran out.

"Hey!" I yelled after her. "What happened to privacy?!"

I wasn't awake enough for a good comeback.

I rolled my eyes and shook my head. Not worth it. Still.

"You'd better sleep with one eye open tonight!" I threatened down the hall.

Okay, yeah yeah. So I had been standing there in my boxer briefs, shirtless, flexing my arms in front of my mirror when she walked in on me.

What do you expect? It's kind of weird but muscles are a pretty big deal at my place. My parents are exercise fanatics. My dad is a gym teacher and a basketball coach, and my mom is a yoga instructor. And Dad is always saying, "Let's see those pipes son," and squeezing my biceps, followed by a big "Yeah!"

After a while, it rubs off.

I don't disclose this to many people voluntarily but my full name is Finnegan Ian Tilley.

And if you noticed my initials, I'll tell you now: Yes they did that on purpose. My parents are both such exercise nuts that they thought it would be cute to have a kid with the initials F.I.T. When I was five, the first thing they did after they registered me for school was call L.L. Bean and order my personalized backpack with my initials. Yikes.

Luckily, fitness is my area. I've read those books about kid detectives who help all their friends find their missing pets, get them out of scams, save the world from blowing up, that kind of thing? I do that, but with exercise. I don't get paid yet, but someday…

Hey, people are making money being 'life coaches' for grown ups. They're basically detectives:

"You can't find time to get your life together and exercise?

Let's look at your schedule.

Stop watching so much t.v. and wasting time.

Take the stairs instead of the elevator.

Walk to work and don't be so lazy!"

That sort of thing.

I think I'd be pretty good at bossing people around and getting paid for it. Why not get a head start?

Case in point: the reason for the text.

My buddy Charlie called me up last night, totally freaked out that his mom is threatening to put him in 'I Can Lose It' (I know – ICLI – sounds icky). It's this weight-watching program.

He was picturing himself trapped in a room

with a bunch of middle-aged women wearing muumuus. I could tell he was upset because his voice went up three octaves. For a big guy, that's a little weird.

I talked him down last night, but his mom probably freaked him out all over again this morning.

I'll admit, Charlie is… hmm, how to say it… chunky. He wasn't always this big. When I first met Charlie a few years ago, he was your average kid, albeit a little big-boned, as they call it.

His family moved here to North Carolina from England right around the time we moved here from Canada. We bonded right away, as we navigated our way through being in a new country together.

You wouldn't think there would be all that many differences between Canada, England, and the United States, but there are a few. Like, Charlie had to get used to calling potato chips 'chips' as opposed to 'crisps' like they do in England. And what he used to call 'chips' are French fries. You get my drift. Growing up in Canada, we got lots of influences from both the U.S. and England, so I was okay, but Charlie had to figure out pretty quickly that no one knew what the heck he was talking about when he said stuff like "I fancy bangers and mash!" (Fancy means to really like or love something. And bangers and mash is sausages and potatoes by the way. I guess it's a real classic in England. And it's good!)

Anyway, back to the size thing. We started out about the same. I was a little skinnier and he was a little more rugged looking, but now Charlie's a pretty big guy. He's also way taller than everyone in my class, even the girls, so that doesn't exactly make him look diminutive. Basically, Charlie looks like a big, roly-poly puppy. On growth hormone.

Anyway. Hmm, speaking of diminutive – brain, that is - I didn't hear my sister's hyena-like laugh anymore. I pulled on shorts and my favorite t-shirt: a classic green Adidas Original.

Ralph was lounging on my bed. He's a three year-old black Labrador retriever and bed hog, and he (no matter what anyone else in the family says) is *my* dog. He's awesome.

"Come on Ralphie," I coaxed. I ambled downstairs as he raced past me.

It was the usual scene: Mom was at the blender, whipping up another concoction, or as she calls it, 'lifestyle smoothie'. Dad was reading the sports section of the newspaper with his mug of coffee, or as he calls it, 'sweet, sweet nectar'.

I don't quite get the coffee addiction frankly. It smells like a cross between the forest floor and a horse barn. But if it takes away the morning crankies, drink up.

Speaking of cranky, my pain-in-the-butt, er I mean, lovely sister was looking at the J Crew catalogue and whining to Mom about buying her yet more clothes while batting her oatmeal muffin back and forth like a soccer ball. Special. I swear, that girl is eleven years old and she's already a clothes hound. Lately she's been on a real grumpy fest too.

"Don't you like the muffins, Fiona? How about

some oatmeal?" I heard my mom ask as I strolled into the kitchen. I heard her grunt something about not being hungry. How can you not be hungry after eight hours in dreamland? I don't get that.

I made my entrance in my (definitely not designer) attire. But my t-shirt and gym shorts were clean and rip free, so that's not bad.

Now, in many families, morning is a pretty chilled out time of day. Everyone is just waking up and getting their sea legs, as it were. Not in my family. My parents can be pretty cool, but they're also a little over the top.

I murmured, "Morning," and braced for it.

My mom spun around, and happy rays just about shot out of her body. "Good morning Sunshine!" she exclaimed, as if me walking in the kitchen was the best surprise ever. (By the way, I'm trying to train her out of the Sunshine thing.)

Then she lunged for me and caught me up in a bear hug, finishing it off with a smoochie, loud kiss, a little too close to my ear. (Eardrum still intact.)

Mental note: Tell Mom to ease off on the protein powder.

Then Dad, whipped closed his paper and boomed, "Morning big guy! How's my guy this morning?"

Since I was still in Mom's bearhug deathgrip, it took me a second or two to respond. Mom loosened the claws and went back to her blender, humming.

I sat down at the table with a soft, "Great Dad". I coughed a little.

"Awesome son!" boomed Dad.

"Fiona, how about some fruit and yogurt then?" Mom was sounding a little desperate. Fiona shook her head.

"Stay out of my room Fifi," I greeted my sister. (I love calling her that. She hates it.)

Then, without even looking up from the catalogue, Fiona piped in, "Are your Grover arms any bigger today?"

Before I could answer, my dad grabbed my arm (see what I mean?), and declared, "Look at those pipes! That's my boy!"

That is my family. Like some kind of wholesome t.v. family… on steroids. Now that I was in middle school, this daily mauling ritual had become just another part of my routine.

I yawned. "How'd the Tar Heels do last night?"

"Easy win," my dad stated proudly. "They could go all the way this year. Again."

Mom placed a glass of her smoothie in front of me, and I thought I heard a low growl.

Dad went to The University of North Carolina here in Chapel Hill. Mom went to Duke. They both ran track. Dad was an awesome basketball player in high school, but track was where he had the most success, so he got a running scholarship.

Basketball is huge here. To say there's a rivalry between Duke and UNC is like saying that nobody really likes Voldemort in Harry Potter. It's a major understatement.

"You know, I think this could be their best basketball team in years," Dad chipped in. Mom made some kind of "tehh!" sound.

Mom's actually from Canada, but I guess she was a pretty good runner too, and got a scholarship to go to university in the good ole U S of A.

My folks met at a Duke - Carolina basketball game, which is pretty funny, considering the rivalry between the two universities. If you look up 'greatest sports rivalries', I can guarantee Duke – Carolina basketball is at the top of the list.

So it must have been fate. I think my folks kind of knew each other through track too, but the teams never mingled. How they ended up going on a date, let alone getting hitched, I'll never know. Lucky they did though. Or I wouldn't be here. I was born in Canada and we lived there for a while. Just call me international man of mystery! (Hmm, or not.)

I've been to quite a few college games and man it's cool. Besides the sheer awesomeness of the hoops, you've got the band, the cheerleaders, the dancers, and the tasty snacks. Everyone wears the school colors. So at home games, it's a sea of Carolina blue.

I love it. In fact, I love all university sports. There's just so much spirit. What I love most is that it's not a money thing for the athletes. They're loyal to their school forever. Anyway, I digress.

I grabbed a muffin and took a satisfying gulp of my smoothie. Yes, blueberry. I gave Mom a thumb's up as I started to devour the muffin. She winked and continued to bop around.

I started to wrap my mind around the day. It was Friday, and I had library and gym today. Not too shabby.

Just then, the doorbell rang. I looked at the clock: eight o'clock on the nose. The only person who shows up with such precision is Charlie.

CHAPTER 2

My mom bounded to the door, almost collid-
ing with Ralph, who was also determined to get
to Charlie first.

"Good morning Charlie," my mom half-called,
half-sang, as she opened the door, shooing Ralph
back.

"Hello Kate," Charlie returned gamely, in his
upper crusty British accent. Then in an Irish accent, "Top o' the mornin' to ya!"

Mom laughed. "Oh Charlie. I love your spirit."

Then he followed her into the kitchen, in all
his Charlie-ness: big grin, messy hair, overloaded
backpack.

He sat down beside Dad as Ralph slobbered all
over him. Charlie slobbered right back. He loves
animals but his dad is allergic. So is his maid.

"Hey Charlie!" Dad boomed. "What's the
good news?"

Meanwhile, Mom, who loves Charlie, brought
him over a glass of smoothie. "Try this. It's good
for your immune system."

Charlie took a slug. "Thank you. This is brilliant!" Then, to Dad: "Blimey, North Carolina really trounced Duke last night, hey?"

Dad nodded approvingly to Charlie before he high-fived him. I heard another guttural sound. Was that Mom seriously growling?

"They'd better watch Duke next game though," Charlie continued, turning to Mom. "If Willis hadn't gotten into foul trouble, it could have been a whole different ball game."

Mom nodded. "Exactly," she agreed. "Just wait," Mom predicted, aimed at Dad, "Blue Devils are going to win it next time."

Talk about the art of the suck up. Did I mention my parents love Charlie? If I didn't have a positive self-image, I'd be a little worried. And he loves them. Charlie hangs out at my place all the time. Most guys our age want some space, but Charlie gets enough space at home. (Literally, his house is humongous.)

Here, he gets a big dose of cozy and in-your-face, and seems to like it. Charlie's like the third kid in this family. Fourth, if you count Ralph.

I'll go out on a limb and tell you something: All of my friends actually like my parents. So do I. I mean, you know how kids either don't get along with the parental units, or just sort of disengage? Everyone seriously thinks my parents are cool. Quirky as heck, but cool.

My folks are pretty good at giving us space when needed, but my friends actually like to hang out, even when they're around. Most of their parents are working all the time, so I guess it's a novel thing. Plus my parents are pretty laid back.

I looked at Charlie. He had a funny expression on his face – the kind he gets when he's going over lines right before a play - part concentration, part stress, part looking like he's holding in a fart.

Charlie downed the last of his smoothie. And I mean downed it. He held his head back so far, trying to get out the last drops that I thought he was going to tip backwards off the chair. Finally he straightened up. "Ready to roll amado hermano?"

I looked at him with raised eyebrows.

"It means 'beloved brother' in Spanish," he said.

"Aww!" That was my mom.

(You may now be imagining Spanish spoken with a proper British accent. Yes, it sounds as weird as you're imagining.)

I got up. "Ohh-kaaay," I returned, tilting my head to the side. "Gee Charlie, I'm touched," I replied a little sarcastically. Truth is, I do love the big lug like a brother. But come on, I've got an image here.

"We're going to Spain for a few days next month with Dad," Charlie added. "I'm studying."

Charlie is a whiz at languages, so I'm sure he'll be pretty bueno at speaking Spanish.

"Muchos coolio," I nodded. Charlie gave me his blank 'are you joking' look.

"Thanks so much for the smoothie Kate," Charlie added as we got up from the table. "It was fantastic."

"You boys walking or riding?" my Dad asked. Dad coaches and teaches at the high school right next to our school, and usually walks or rides his bike also. But he knows how to give me space. Plus, I'm sure he has to get his head together before dealing with all those seventeen year olds.

"We're walking Dad," I returned solemnly. "We've got something important to talk about."

Charlie's voice, obviously reminded of his problem, went sky high again.

"Have a good one!" he half-called, half-shrieked at my family. It even made Fiona look up from her catalogue.

CHAPTER 3

We meandered down the sidewalk, me dribbling my basketball with one hand and sipping my smoothie (in my personalized F.I.T. thermos – see what I mean) with the other. Charlie filled me in.

His mom took him to the doctor yesterday for his annual check-up, and once he stepped on the scale, it was downhill from there.

"I knew it was trouble when Doctor Jones gave me his two tone 'hmm-mm'," Charlie recounted. "So then he gets out a chart and starts telling Mom my BMI is too high. So I say, 'Well Doc, let's write me out a prescription and take care of it shall we?'"

I looked at Charlie, nodding. His voice had gone up a few notes if that was possible. It cracked.

"It's okay man," I soothed. "Simmer down and tell me what happened next."

Charlie cleared his throat. He was sweating. "Can we slow down a little here mate? What is this, a race?"

Now that we were effectively at turtle pace, he continued into a babble. "So then Mother tells me that I'm not Bugs Bunny, and don't call him Doc – not a great time to push the etiquette training. Then Doc Jones said that BMI is a measure of how much you weigh compared to your height, something about weight-related health, and if BMI is too high, it's bad for your health. And mine is too (and again, the voice accompanying here) high! So basically I have too much fat for my height! Can you believe it? I mean, what do I have to be? Six foot five?!"

I stowed my thermos and rubbed my chin with my non-dribbling hand. Then I rubbed my ear. Charlie's voice was high enough to break glass.

"Did he tell your mom to take you to I.C.L.I.," I asked, "or was it Beatrice's idea?"

(Beatrice is Charlie's mom. And yes, we're all scared of her.)

"Her all the way," Charlie told me. "She was so very embarrassed that her son would be," using his bunny ear air quotations, "overweight."

I nodded, processing what he was telling me.

Charlie shook his head. "I mean, she's the one who feeds me! Well, she pays Alice to feed me!"

By the way, Alice is Charlie's chef. Did I mention that he's rich? I should clarify that: Charlie's stinking rich.

"What did your dad say?" I asked, continuing to gather info. "I mean, he's not exactly a small guy either."

"Dad's away on business for a week or two," Charlie said a little bitterly.

Charlie's dad is a super formal dude. I mean, I know people from England (case in point: Charlie), and besides the cool accent and some interesting words for stuff, they're just like us.

Not Charlie's dad. Mr. Bienenstock is like something out of a James Bond movie. I've even heard him say, "Bienenstock. Charles Bienenstock." (Okay, not the same ring as James Bond, but still super intimidating.) And he's a pretty imposing figure at six foot three or so. He's not fat but he is a big man.

"Regardless," Charlie rambled, "It doesn't help when your doctor is an ex-NCAA All-American sprinter. I mean, the chap still has muscles bulging under his stethoscope. Of course I'd look a little pudgy by comparison!"

We were almost at school now, and I thought Charlie was going to hyperventilate. He's definitely a guy who wears his heart on his sleeve, and his worries too.

He stopped and faced me, and I stopped dribbling. My ball that is.

"And another thing, he did about a five second calculation. Maybe he hit the wrong button. Plus I'm just about to have a growth spurt any day. I mean, I can't help how tall I am. That shouldn't be an issue with my weight! Plus I'm big-boned!"

Hmm, Doc Jones is my doctor too. He's a friend of my folks so I know him pretty well. I call him Davis. He's a pretty smart guy, so I doubt he made a mistake. But it's possible. As for Charlie going through a growth spurt, if he does, he's going to be getting calls from NBA scouts. The big-boned thing? Maybe.

"It's okay," I reassured him. "I'll look into it. We have library this morning, and if I don't find anything, I'll call Dad."

Charlie took a deep breath and nodded. "Thanks Finn."

I had one last question: "How much time do you have?"

"The next meeting is on Tuesday," Charlie told me grimly. He stopped and put his hand on my shoulder. "Godspeed."

I didn't know what Godspeed meant, but I'd heard it in a few movies and it sounded melodramatic but kind of cool. Did I mention Charlie's in drama? He's actually a really good actor.

(Okay, just looked it up. Godspeed means 'good fortune' or 'success'. Cool.)

"Hey! Finn, Charlie!" It was Chris, my other best friend.

By the way, just so I don't give you the wrong mental picture right off the bat, Chris is a girl.

Christina Rosa Maria Ruez (now you get the nickname) is one of the coolest girls in school. We've been together since grade three, where we shared a mat at reading time. I think I had a little crush on her in grade four. At some point, we became great friends. Chris is one of those girls who can do anything. She's really good at sports, plays the violin, and she's smart as a whip. (Oh crap, that's something my grampa would say.)

Chris half ran, half skipped over to us, with her usual crazy and boundless energy. I took out my smoothie again and took a slug, finishing it off.

"Hey Chris," I said, trying to inject a little energy into it.

"Hey Finn!" Chris pumped back. And to Charlie, "Hey Big Guy!"

Hmm, wrong choice of words. Only I could hear his whimper.

The bell rang and Charlie and I dragged ourselves up the Stairs of Doom while Chris bounded up them two at a time.

Okay okay, the 'Stairs of Doom' thing: I don't really hate school. It's mostly just a façade.

I mean seriously, how many middle school guys do you know that go around saying, "Ooh I love school so much! I'm SO looking forward to school!"

Exactly: none.

Even if you love school – which I'm not saying I do – you have to be cool about it.

Also:

Favorite subject? Gym. Always gym. Even if it's also math. (I'm more of an English guy myself.)

Best thing about school? Recess. Not even debatable.

Again, I digress.

We walked into class, as Ms. MacMurray, our homeroom teacher, got up from her desk and welcomed us to a new day. I took a deep breath. It sounded like I was sighing, but I wasn't really. Mom would call it a cleansing breath. (I can't believe I just said that.)

Again, not that I'd admit this loudly, but I kind of like this part of the morning: walking in, seeing my classmates, wondering what's ahead. Maybe a surprise art class, maybe a fire drill. Who knows? This morning we had library just before recess. It would be a little quiet time with the books before we could let loose on the playground. I could start my research into Charlie's little problem.

"Good morning everyone," rang out Ms. Mac. "Nice to have you here. How are you all today?" (See what I mean? Just a nice way to start the day.)

We all mumbled, so a collective "guddd" came out. So I guess we were all good.

And our 'gud' day started.

CHAPTER 4

A little while later, I was sitting in the library, my nose in a book while Charlie breathed over my shoulder.

"Nothing here," I whispered to Charlie, as I closed one book and opened another.

"There's got to be something," breathed Charlie urgently. I turned my head to look at him, almost touching noses.

"Not helping," I stated. He backed off a little and I went back to scanning the book.

"Sorry mate, sorry," he said. "I just don't know what I should do."

He slumped back in the chair beside me, putting his head in his hands. Then he leaned back and did kind of a back arch/slump into the back of his chair, shaking his head at the ceiling. He turned his face toward me.

Sometimes he really cracks me up without meaning to. I looked at Charlie and leaned toward him. "Here's a crazy idea," I advised. "Since we're in the library, why don't you (I paused for dramatic effect) get yourself a book."

"Oh yeah. Right," he chuckled. Then he got in my face again. "I'm just so bloody stressed, I don't know if I can concentrate."

I smiled at Charlie, that tense smile that I've seen Mom use on me when she's really miffed and trying to hold it together. "Charlie. Help me help you." (I heard that line in 'Jerry Maquire', a sports movie. I like it. Must use again.)

(Charlie obviously didn't see the movie.) He looked at me blankly. "Huh?"

"Help me help you," I repeated, now using my hands to gesture. "Go look in the phys. ed. section for any books that might have something about BMI or weight."

Charlie straightened up. "Right. Yeah," he muttered, as he walked toward the shelves.

Within one minute, I heard laughter from the stacks. It was the Russell twins, Molly and Maggie, goofing around with Charlie. They belong to the same country club as Charlie's family, and their house is almost as big.

Maggie and Molly are identical. The only way to tell them apart is the scar on Molly's chin from a playground accident when she was a preschooler. Think: Molly had a fall-y and you remember who's who. They're both pretty fun. A little snobby sometimes, but they're nice to me.

A little more twittering (hopefully the girls and not Charlie), followed by our librarian's voice. "Charles. No fooling around during library. Pick out a book please," scolded Ms. Bowdon.

"Sorry Ms. Bowdon," Charlie purred back.

"Did I ever tell you what a stellar librarian you are?"

"It's okay Charlie," she replied, in her I-know-you're-trying-to-charm-me tone. Yes, she was instantly charmed.

"I mean, you have a gift," he continued from somewhere in the stacks. I looked across at Chris and rolled my eyes. Chris pretended to throw up. We both laughed.

Ms. Bowdon walked out of the stacks toward us. "Less chatting and more looking Charlie," she followed up, in her you-just-went-too-far-in-the-suck-up-department tone, shaking her head.

Ms. Bowdon is the polar opposite of what you think a librarian should look like. Whenever I read a book with a librarian character in it, they're always old, dowdy, and stern but caring. Okay, Ms. Bowdon has the stern caring part, but definitely not dowdy! I don't know why I never noticed before this year, but Ms. Bowdon is actually cool. And, I can't believe I'm saying this, but she's hot. You know what I mean. She's still pretty old, thirty I think. But she dresses like a kid. Super hip. And the best is, she drives this old Jaguar! She told me one time that she always wanted to have a Jag, and she bought it second-hand and cheap, relatively speaking. Plus, her brother's a mechanic, so he helps keep it running. Any girl who makes cars a priority is all right with me!

As Ms. Bowdon approached, I raised my hand.

"Hey Finn, what's happening?" she asked, sitting down beside me. She smelled like oranges.

I showed her the book I was looking at. "I'm

trying to find something on BMI but I can't really find something to explain it. I just keep finding references to it."

"BMI as in body mass index?" she asked, looking at me with her chin on her hand, her hair falling over her shoulder.

"Yeah," I replied, blinking a couple of times to concentrate. "I guess so. The weight thing." Of course all this would have been way easier if Charlie had just asked her for a reference himself, instead of being Mr. Suck Up. I guess he was embarrassed, and I understand that. I looked up to see him sneaking a piece of chocolate into his mouth.

Ms. Bowdon flipped to the back of the book. "Sometimes it's listed under BMI and sometimes under body mass index," she said. She picked up another book. "You're looking in the right places Finn," she said. "There's just not a lot of information in these books. I'll tell you, your dad will have all this stuff in his books and papers."

Ms. Bowdon knows my dad through school, teachery circles. And Mom said she goes to her yoga class.

"But we'll get a start on it." She wiggled her finger toward the computers. "Follow me." And like a puppy dog, I followed.

CHAPTER 5

I plunked down at the computer, and Ms. Bowdon sat down beside me.

"I would search body mass index first, instead of using the abbreviation," she advised. "Why the interest?"

I typed in the words, then looked at her. "It's for a friend," I said quietly. "His BMI is too high and he's kind of freaked out. And embarrassed."

Ms. Bowdon nodded. "Oh. I see," she whispered. She looked at the screen. "Here we go," she said. I looked at the screen as she read it out loud.

"Body mass index, or BMI. An anthropometric index to indicate health risks associated with body weight and composition."

Ms. Bowdon turned to me. My eyes were wide.

"You lost me at anth-ro-po-," I said tensely.

"Yes, wow, that's a little complicated sounding, isn't it?" she returned. "Well, let's break it down, she continued calmly. "Anthropometric means 'body measurement', by the way."

"Cool."

"Yeah," she continued. "It comes from Greek. 'Anthropo' meaning human, and 'metric' meaning measurement."

She seemed a little more excited about that fact than I was.

She got out a piece of paper and wrote down 'body mass index'. "An index is like a guide or a chart with information. Your body mass is basically how much you weigh."

She turned back to the keyboard and typed a few words.

"Okay, here it is. Yes. Body mass index, or BMI is a measure of body weight compared to height. They use a calculation to get your BMI and then see where it fits in a chart. If it's too low, you may be underweight. If it's too high, you may be overweight. You might have too much body fat, and you're at risk."

"For what?" I asked.

Ms. Bowdon flicked her hair back. "Oh gosh, there are a lot of health problems related to being really overweight. Diabetes and stress on your joints, like the knees. Being very overweight can lead to issues later on, like heart disease." She paused, like she was choosing her words carefully, then plowed onward. "Plus, some kids have self-esteem issues. You know, they don't feel so confident if they're quite overweight. Maybe they're embarrassed, like your friend. That shouldn't be an issue, but sometimes it is. The list goes on."

Suddenly, I was feeling a little stressed for

Charlie. I didn't want him to be sick or feel bad. This was getting personal.

I looked at Ms. Bowden and shrugged. "But why do some kids have high BMI? I mean," I trailed off, shrugging again. My shoulders had become ear warmers.

"A high BMI can be related to sedentary behaviour," she said. Off my look, she added, "Sedentary means you're just sitting or laying around all the time. It's inactivity. That's one factor. But there's a lot more to BMI, Finn. We're just scratching the surface," she concluded.

Ms. Bowdon looked at the clock. My classmates were rustling around like a bunch of cattle, closing books, dumping scraps of paper in the garbage, getting ready to move on. Library was almost over. Charlie looked over at me hopefully. I turned back to Ms. Bowdon.

"Okay. Here's the equation for BMI," she said. She pointed to the screen:

BMI = weight (kg) / height (m^2)

I looked at it. "Whoa," I blurted. Instant mind blank.

She laughed, then put her chin on her hand and looked at me thoughtfully. "If it's for a friend whose BMI is too high, you may also want to look up 'weight control'," she said quietly.

"Yeah," I said nodding. (So much for sparklingly intelligent responses.)

"And I would suggest he or she talk to someone about it," she added. "Weight can be kind of a touchy issue."

She slid her pencil over her ear and smiled.

The cattle continued to rustle.

"I can run through this now with you," she said. "But I don't want you to miss any of your recess."

I straightened up. "Yeah," I replied. (Again, where were all the other words in my repertoire!)

I felt a little guilty. I mean, Charlie's my buddy, but a guy's got to blow off some steam. This could wait a little while.

Just then the bell rang, and you'd think they had just announced free pizza in the gym or something. Pa-toing! Everyone rushed out.

"Like I mentioned Finn," Ms. Bowdon said as we stood up, "your dad will have all this information. In fact, he'll probably have better stuff." She smiled. "Can you touch base with me and let me know if I can do anything else to help?"

I nodded. Ms. Bowden really is the coolest librarian. She doesn't talk down to you or make it seem like a hassle to help you.

I grabbed my books. "Thanks a lot Ms. Bowdon, I really appreciate it," I said earnestly.

She winked at me. "Anytime Finn," she smiled.

Ahhh.

CHAPTER 6

I jogged out into the schoolyard to join my class. They were hanging out around the four-square and green recreation area. (In case you're wondering, yes, it's really a playground.)

A lot of middle schools just have pavement, a basketball court, and maybe a bit of grass, so students just go outside and flake out or stand around and do nothing, but they did some research and found that if you have some kind of playground, even teenagers will be more active. The old 'if you build it, they will come' deal. (That's a line from another great sports movie, 'Field of Dreams'. The farmer actually bulldozes his corn and builds a baseball field!)

In our case, it was 'if you build it, they will get off their butts'. It works. I've even seen college students playing on the structures on the weekends.

Our green playground is pretty cool. Last year, our old playground was just about falling down, so the Parent Teacher Association decided to put in a new one as a big community project. This new one is all natural. They say that's better for kids and teenagers, and we can concentrate better after hanging out in 'nature' as opposed to on metal and concrete. I'll buy it.

There's one older set of metal monkey bars. (But let's face it, monkey bars are classic. You cannot just be around them without wanting to climb or hang on them.) Other than that, it's mostly logs and climbing trees, and some funky climbing equipment. There's a huge sand court for beach volleyball, and a garden. We actually get class time to come out and tend the garden. So by the end of the year, we'll supposedly eat what we've grown. (That could be a little scary but I'm open to anything.) My favorite thing is the obstacle course made out of logs and boulders. There's also a 'green track' as they call it, so kids can walk around while they talk, as opposed to just standing or sitting around to gab. The 'green track' cracks us up, because it's just a path. But I guess they try to name things to make them sound more enticing.

As I approached my class, I scanned the scene. What would I want to do first? Some of the kids were running around, some were climbing, playing with a ball, a few of the girls were walking around on the little path, talking and giggling (scratch that off the list). A couple of kids were checking out the garden.

Charlie was reclining on a log with a group of kids over by The Art Part. This area is pretty cool. When they re-did the playground, they put up these huge boards. They're like big canvasses for art, only they're more like white boards. You can draw anything you want and either wipe it off with a wet rag, or just let the rain wash it away. It's supposed to 'encourage creativity and quiet reflection'.

Last year, they took the boards down for a while after one guy drew something that encouraged his suspension and a quiet essay on what's appropriate. But they gave it another chance and it's been amazing seeing some of the cool drawings and inspirational messages. Some of my classmates are really talented.

"Hey Finn!"

I looked over. It was a couple of my friends, Xavier and Tom.

Xavier and I have a kind of bond over our names: We usually call him Xav (pronounced 'Zave') and of course I always go by Finn. But on the first day of school, we always get called by our full names: Xavier Aloysius and Finnigan Ian. Everyone chuckles, and we look at each other and shake our heads. It's become a tradition.

Xavier waved me over. He's a big jock in our class. He's one of those guys who's pretty good at everything he tries, but he also works like crazy, and you have to respect that. He's insanely good at hoops (which I know is stereotypically African American, which Xavier is) and he's a really tough competitor. Plus he's a good sport, fun to play sports and games with, you know? We call him mini Andrew Wiggins (an awesome basketball player and, ahem, Canadian), because he looks like him, and he acts like him. Xavier's a class act.

Xav and Tom were on the grass with a soccer ball so I headed in their direction.

"Hey guys," I called as I jogged over.

Tom's another cool guy in our class. He also moved here a few years ago from Canada, so he's a fellow Canuck, but he never played hockey either. (Yes, that's something that everyone assumes all Canadian guys do.)

Tom's one of those guys that's also natural athlete. In gym, whenever we learn a new skill, wham! He's got it. I can tell it drives some of the guys nuts, partly because he's so casual about it. He's just not a competitive guy. We play tennis together and he's awesome, but he doesn't get all crazy aggressive like a few of the guys do. He's just happy to be hanging out. He's one of those guys who always has a smile on his face.

"Come and kick around with us," offered Tom. He kicked the ball to me.

"Where were you?" asked Xavier. I kicked the ball back.

"I was looking up something in the library," I returned. "You guys ever heard of BMI?"

They both shook their heads. "Is it a company?" Tom asked. We were getting some nice passes with the soccer ball.

"Nah. It stands for body mass index," I said.

We stopped for a second. "It sounds like something aliens would do in a movie when they abduct people," Xav shot back. Then, in a funny voice, "Come here earthling, we must assess your body mass index with our butt probe scanner." We laughed.

Tom added, "Yeah, it sounds a little creepy, Finn. Why are you interested in that?"

"It's for Charlie," I confided. "It's kind of like how much you weigh and if it's healthy or too little or too much."

"Oh," they both said knowingly, in kind of a dismal tone.

"Don't say anything to him about it though," I added.

The guys nodded. "Yeah, no problem," Tom agreed.

We looked over at Charlie, still reclining, drinking a can of something fizzy and having a snack. He didn't look real worried right now.

And since even detectives need to blow off steam once in a while, I let it go for now and made some massively awesome kicks.

CHAPTER 7

Later on, after lunch, we had gym. Like I said, favorite subject for most people. Not Charlie.

Maybe it's the laps we always have to run to warm up. Maybe it's the fact that he has never been able to charm our teachers. I don't know. But walking into the gym always seems to give Charlie hives.

It doesn't help to have Alan in our class. Alan is almost as big as Charlie, but without the gentle exterior.

It's not like Alan's a bully in the classic sense. More like a blowhard. He's just kind of intense and won't shut up, a guy who thinks he's all that and a bag of chips. It's bad enough to be good at something and brag to everyone else. But when you're mediocre and cocky, that's crap. Alan's never been athletic. Just big and in your face.

We half-walked, half-ran onto the bleachers, Charlie lagging behind as usual, as if being in the gym for that forty seconds less than the rest of us would actually make a difference.

Ms. Devereau stood before us in her usual 'Sheba, Queen of the Jungle' stance, feet shoulder width apart, hands on hips, surveying us.

Must she be so intense? As usual, her shorts and t-shirt were too tight. Gross.

Yes, she's our gym teacher, but we love gym despite her. I'm sure she means well. Maybe.

Joining her was her student teacher for the year, Mr. Harris. He's got potential, but why we have to call the guy Mr. Harris, I do not know. This guy looks like he's in grade ten. Dude's not even shaving yet.

When Mr. Harris stepped out, a few of the girls twittered, and I don't mean getting out their iPhone and sending a tweet, I mean actually putting their hands in front of their mouths and giggling like schoolgirls. Even though they are schoolgirls. You get my point. I think every girl in the class has a crush on him.

Mr. Harris whispered something to Ms. Devereau and she twittered too. Yes, she spends most gym classes flirting with the guy.

The noise level went up and we started goofing around. The class was getting restless and she took the cue.

"Today, we're going to play volleyball," Ms. Devereau announced, and we all cheered. (Except Charlie. The only time he ever cheered in gym was when we did jazz dancing… Which was way more fun than you would think, once you got past the embarrassment. And funny, if you had seen us doing the steps.)

Five minutes later, we were serving, bumping,

and volleying. I was on a court with Tom, Alan, and Molly. Molly, as usual, had this fully coordinated outfit: t-shirt, gym skort (that kooky shorts/skirt combo), little socks with matching pom-poms, and color-coordinated ribbon in her hair. Man, that seems like a lot of work.

We were in a groove, the volleyball sailing back and forth over the net, when I looked over to see Charlie shaking out his hand as if he had hurt it.

Then BOOM, I got a volleyball, hard, on the side of the head.

Molly, who was on my side, rushed over. "Are you okay Finn?" she asked sweetly.

Meanwhile, Alan was laughing hysterically. "Pay attention Finnigan," he laughed.

I shook my head, imagining a few birds flying circles around my head, with a few stars thrown in.

"Hey Alan, that's not funny man," Tom said, sounding miffed. "You saw that Finn was distracted, and you belted it." Like I say, Tom's a good, fair guy.

Alan shrugged indifferently.

"I'm good," I said, blinking a couple of times, then said to Alan, "Not cool man."

He still had that stupid grin on his face.

I heard Ms. Devereau tell Charlie to "sit out then", her tone just this side of exasperated, and I looked to see him walking off, still shaking his hand.

"Switch!" yelled Ms. Devereau and we all moved one position. Now Tom and I were across from Alan and Molly.

Molly served the ball, nice and smoothly over the net.

Alan looked over as Charlie sat down on the bleachers. The ball floated over to me and I set it up for Tom to hit.

Calling out to no one in particular, Alan piped up, "Hey, why does Charlie get to beach himself over there?"

I cringed for Charlie. You could only tell Alan to shut his trap so many times. Sometimes you just had to ignore him.

"Pay attention Alan," Ms. Devereau called back.

SMASH! Tom blasted it. Right in Alan's face.

"Oh sorry Alan," Tom called casually. "My bad. You okay champ?"

"Yeah yeah, just serve," he said to all of us, clearly fuming.

Tom backed up toward me and put his hand out behind him for a low five, which I returned. Truth is, I was surprised. Tom's the most non-aggressive guy I know (tying with Charlie). But he's also a really loyal friend. I guess loyalty won out today. Sometimes Alan just needs to be put in his place.

Speaking of in his place: Charlie had successfully gotten out of most of gym, again. Did he always do this? No. Way back, he didn't. He used to like gym class.

It should make you feel good to come and run around and play games. But as we walked out and Charlie joined us, the expression on his face said relief with a capital R. The rest of his body, kind of stooped, with his shoulders slumped, just looked bummed out.

Tom meanwhile was a little pleased with himself. "Liked the 'champ' bit," Xavier said under his breath.

"Oh, after that (raising his voice) accidental hit?" Tom winked back. "Yeah thanks, I thought it was a nice touch."

We were all laughing, except Charlie who frankly looked a little miserable.

Then the most well-meaning words from Xavier:

"You okay big guy?"

I had to get back to work – and quick.

CHAPTER 8

After school, Charlie had a piano lesson and Chris had taekwondo. This was an off day for me so I walked over to Dad's office.

Like I said, since the high school is pretty much next door to my school, it's a matter of walking about fifty yards and crossing the sports fields. Dad's office is right beside the gym.

I walked into the auditorium entrance, where the gym and stage are. They know me here, so everyone's always pretty nice. I guess no one wants to mess with the basketball coach's kid either. They might land themselves a few extra burpees! (Just kidding.)

I waved to the vice-principal, Ms. Bailey, as she rushed past me with a stack of booklets. She waved back. "How are you Finn?" she called.

"Great Ms. Bailey, how are you?" I returned. (Mom is a stickler for me using someone's name when I talk to him or her. I have to admit, it does score points.)

"Rushed, as usual Finn! I'm late for a meeting.

Nice to see you," she sang back. And she speed-walked down the hall.

I poked my head in the gym. Ah, as expected, the girls' volleyball team was practicing. Not to sound cocky, but these girls love me.

I walked along the wall toward Dad's office. The volleyball team was gathered around Dad, getting instructions for their next drill I guess.

Dad isn't the regular volleyball coach. He helps out sometimes when Lois, the head coach, can't be there. (Like I said, Dad was Mr. Sports when he was a kid, so he played everything and he's good at everything. No pressure!)

Dad's a health and physical education teacher, but his official job here is head basketball coach. He teaches a few P.E. classes too, and helps out at track practices here and there, but his main gig is hoops.

Sports are pretty big here. The high school has turned out some good players, so sometimes university recruiters come to games or meets. Dad knows some of the great university coaches of all time. I've met a few basketball coaches. They're kind of semi-famous.

When we met Coach K from Duke, Mom was a little star struck but he was pretty chilled out. Nice guy.

I got to hang out (on ironclad promise of exceptionally good behavior) once when Coach Roy Williams from The University of North Carolina (UNC) met with a player and his mom at our place. He's such a cool guy, really down to earth.

Anyway, one of the girls spotted me and waved,

then gestured to my dad that I was here. I waved and pointed toward his office. Dad flashed me the 'okay' sign as all the girls turned around and saw me. I got a chorus of "Hi Finn!"

"Hi Girls," I called out. "Work hard!"

They looked at each other and I heard "so cute" from a few of them. Well that's a little embarrassing. I'm not trying to be cute, I'm trying to motivate!

I dropped my backpack and had a seat in Dad's chair. For an office, his is pretty cool, even though it's a little small. Real estate agents would call it 'cozy'. There are lots of sports books, some cool motivational posters, plus all his snacks.

I picked up last month's *Men's Health* magazine that was sitting on Dad's desk, and flipped through it. Hmm, there were some healthy recipes for weekend cooking and grilling.

There was a pile of books in the corner. They all had food on the cover. I got up and sifted through them.

They were diet books!

One had an assortment of veggies on the cover, and said *Meat No More*. One had a big burger on the cover and was called *The Meat Lovers' Guide to Life*. One had a bunch of juices and the title was *Squeeze It Out of You*.

What?

Oh man, if you read all these, you'd only be left with water!

I realized I was hungry.

I swiveled around and opened Dad's mini-fridge. Energy drinks, some cheese, a few apples.

Nothing was ringing my bell. I slid open his snack drawer. Bingo. Granola bars. I grabbed one and swiveled around to the bookshelf. Sometimes you get good info the old-fashioned way: looking in a book.

Right below the 'IF IT IS TO BE, IT IS UP TO ME' poster (see what I mean by motivational), I spotted a book that looked good.

Weight Issues for Young People. I got up and pulled the book, opening it to the table of contents. Hmm, not promising. The chapter headings were a little touchy-feely for my liking: 'The Mind Body Connection' (huh?), 'Self-esteem and Weight' (uh uh), 'Loving Yourself, Not Your Fridge' (hurl-a-rama).

Next!

I put the book back and perused the shelves again. Ah, *Physical Fitness Assessment*. Bingo. I went to the index this time. Yes! A whole section on body mass index.

I started reading. I only got about three paragraphs in, when Cassie stuck her head in.

Cassie's one of the seniors, and the captain, on the volleyball team, and she's good. I mean really good. She's going to university next year, and Dad says she'll get a full-ride scholarship. The university will pay for everything if she plays for them.

Sweet deal if you ask me.

Cassie also comes over to hang out with us here and there. When I was a kid, she used to babysit, but now she only comes over if Mom and Dad are going to something at dinnertime or super late. She'll come and help with supper and hang out, more like a family friend. We usually watch classic movies together. Cassie's pretty cool. Plus she makes a mean pizza.

"Hey Finn, what's up?" Cassie greeted me as she stepped in.

I swiveled around. "Hey Cassie," I breezed back. "How was practice?"

"Awesome," she said, pumped. "The team is really together this year." She leaned over me. "What are you reading? Is it for school?"

I waved my hand toward the book. "I'm checking out body mass index," I informed her. "You know my buddy Charlie?" I asked.

She nodded and smiled. (Charlie has a huge and very obvious crush on Cassie, so every time she's over at the house, he makes an excuse to come over.)

I continued, "His BMI is too high and he's all freaked out. Frankly, I never even heard of it before today."

Cassie looked at the book I was reading. "Wow. You're a good friend Finn."

I leaned back and gave her my innocent grin. "I know."

"And modest too," she joked back. "Anyway, we learned about BMI in my Healthy Lifestyle class," she continued. "It's just your weight compared to your height. In fact, I did a project on body composition and weight control. It's pretty straightforward."

"Body composition?" I cocked my head to the side like Ralph does.

"Body composition is literally 'what your body

is composed, or made up, of". You know, bone, muscle, organs, fat. BMI is a way of estimating if you have a healthy body composition."

Cassie flipped a page. "Do you have his height and weight?"

I raised my eyebrows. "Uh, no," I admitted. I grabbed my notebook and wrote:

GET CHARLIE'S HEIGHT AND WEIGHT.

Cassie grabbed a pen. "Let's figure out your BMI then," she said, motioning me to stand up. "Come over here and let's see how tall you are."

I got up and stood next to the height marker on Dad's wall as Cassie peered over the top of my head. "Wow Finn," she exclaimed. "Five foot three! What are your parents feeding you?"

Cassie led me to the scale. "Step on please, sir!"

I grinned despite myself. Cassie cracks me up, and we have a pretty cool relationship. She gets it that I'm not a kid anymore. I took off my sneakers and stepped on.

"You're in the triple digits Finn! A hundred and one big ones."

I raised my eyebrows and shrugged. Truth is, most of my friends have had these major growth spurts, and I'm still waiting. So I'm not exactly the most physically intimidating guy in my class right now.

Just then Dad stepped into the doorway of his office. "Hey guys," he greeted us.

There was something bothering me. I had to ask. "You trying to shed a few pounds Dad?"

He looked at me quizzically. I pointed to the pile of diet books. He started laughing.

"If I followed all of those, I'd be down to water!"

(What's that old saying? Great minds think alike?)

"Don't worry Finn, I'm just reading them for interest," he said. "Some of these books get a lot of hype in the media, and sometimes students ask me about them."

I nodded. "Oh, I get it."

"It's actually quite fascinating to read them," Dad went on. "Some are pretty well thought out, like the Mediterranean approach where you eat lots of tomatoes, good fats like avocado and olive oil, and that kind of thing. But some are way out there, and cut out a ton of healthy foods."

"I read about one that only lets you eat foods that are chartreuse," Cassie said, laughing.

Dad started laughing too. Then something caught his attention in the gym.

He looked over his shoulder and called back, "You looking for Cassie? She's in here."

Dad stepped in, toward the books, grinning. "I read that one a while ago too. That was a piece of work."

I looked at them both, unimpressed.

"Can somebody please enlighten me here? Shar tooth? What the heck?"

"It's pronounced shar-troos. Believe it or not Finn, it's a color," Cassie said, still chuckling.

"It's like a light greeny yellowish."

"Gross." (I know, not very eloquent of me, but it was the first word I thought of.) "So, you can only eat stuff that's yellowy greenish," I challenged.

"According to this latest craze," Cassie replied, shaking her head.

"It's really important to focus on foods that are healthy, and to be aware of any allergies or sensitivities," Dad finished. "But I'm not a fan of completely knocking out major food groups if you don't have to. I think it's all about balance."

Cassie gave a big nod in my direction.

I was just processing that when a couple of the volleyball girls peaked in. "Hey," they chimed in unison.

"Hey, guys, I'll just be a minute," Cassie said. "We're just checking Finn's BMI."

The girls stepped in with a little "oh" between them. What were they, the backup singers for Lady Gaga?

I stepped off the scale. This was turning into a veritable party. I looked over at Dad who seemed to be loving this. "Now where is my calculator?" he wondered out loud, opening his drawer. He rummaged through a bunch of junk for a jiffy, then found it and handed it to Cassie.

"Thanks Coach. Okay Finn," Cassie said, taking charge. "Here's the body mass index equation." Then to Dad, "Can I use the whiteboard Coach?"

(* Just to cut in here, if you were to read all of Cassie's calculations right now, your brain would go to jelly like mine did. If you're interested, I wrote some stuff down in my notebook at the back. And I'll have some info on my website.)

(Oh yeah, if you see more *italics* in the next page or so? That's me zoning out. Sorry!)

Dad nodded and she wrote:

BMI = weight (kg) / height (m²)

"This looks complicated but it's really not," assured Cassie. It's just a way of looking at your height compared to your weight to see if it's within a healthy range."

As Cassie wrote, she said, "So, your weight is 101 pounds. Your height is 5 feet 3 inches. We just have to convert it so it fits the equation."

(I wonder what's for supper?)

"See Finn?"

And I zoned back in.

We have to change pounds to kilograms," Cassie continued. "Then we have to change inches to centimeters."

(I should check out those new tennis shoes this weekend. How to get Mom to buy them is another question. Hmm. Ah, appeal to Dad.)

I watched Cassie write. Or should I say, I watched her arm fly around on the whiteboard as she chucked numbers up there like crazy. I'm glad we don't have chalkboards anymore or she'd be standing in a cloud of dust.

(Chartreuse. That sounds like an opera, not a color!)

She rambled as she wrote:

"101 pounds divided by 2.2 to get kilograms… You change meters to centimeters… just move your decimal over…"

(I should see if Chris wants to catch that new action movie when it comes out next week. What's it called again?)

Cassie turned around. "You're a little over a meter and a half tall Finn," she smiled. She must have noticed my wide-eyed look of terror because she grinned and added brightly, "Almost done!"

(I'm still hungry.)

She turned back to the board and her hand started popping more numbers on the board like it was possessed. Was she actually enjoying this?

(Yeah, Dad will totally get me those tennis shoes. My ankle's been a little sore anyway. I need them. He's the softie with that. All I have to do is limp around a little, then tell him my old tennis shoes are wearing out because I'm moving around on the court so much. He'll love that.)

"So BMI is your weight in kilograms over your height in meters, squared," she mumbled as the numbers started to blur before my eyes. "All we have to do is…"

(I could go for a pizza right now.)

Still muttering, she continued. "So we get 18.5," she trailed off.

(Oh man, pizza with pineapple and green olives. Sounds gross but it's that perfect combination of salty and sweet.)

Cassie turned around and looked at me proudly. "So, your BMI is 18 and a half!"

I snapped out of it. "Huh?" I said blankly.

I think I still had that stunned look on my face, because everyone broke out laughing. Cassie ruffled my hair. Usually not allowed, but she had just put in a good chunk of time showing me this insane calculation (even though I zoned out), so I smiled and let it go.

"Were you even listening," she said smiling.

I shrugged. "Cass, you know me and math," I said sheepishly.

"Thinking about those new tennis shoes again?" she popped back, winking.

"Well, my ankle has been a little sore lately," I said in my most innocent voice, glancing at Dad. "I think my old shoes are worn out."

Dad snapped to attention. "Really Finn?" (Yes!)

I nodded at Dad and rubbed my ankle for good measure. "I think it's starting to affect my game."

Those shoes were as good as mine.

"We can't have that buddy," Dad said gently. "Let's go this weekend."

Oh yeah!

Cassie ruffled my hair again. It was only then that I noticed Carolina (yes, the girls' tennis team captain and, the most awesome girl ever!) walk by the office. She saw me, mid hair ruffle, and smiled!

Ugh, she probably thought I looked like a little kid. Hmm, on second thought, maybe she thought I looked cool, hanging out with the girls' volleyball team. Okay, no damage-

"Hey Carolina!" Ergh, it was Cassie. "What's up?"

Carolina backed up and appeared in the doorway with a hopper of tennis balls. "Hey Cass, hey guys, what are you all up to?"

The girls/backup singers chorused, "Hey CC."

(CC is what Carolina's friends call her. Talk about cute.)

"Hey CC," Cassie breezed. "We're showing Finn here what body mass index is. You know Finn, right? Finn, Carolina."

Just keep your cool, I thought to myself as she focused on me. Just keep your cool.

"Hi Finn. I've seen you at the tennis center," she said, smiling. "You're good."

"Hi. Uh, thanks Carolina," I replied. (How boring! Ugh!)

"Call me CC," she returned, in that cute sporty voice of hers.

I put one hand up in a casual thumb's up while reaching behind me with the other hand, to lean nonchalantly against Dad's desk.

I somehow forgot that it wasn't near me.

So, instead of giving a modest yet witty response, I lost my balance and went flying backwards onto the floor.

"Whoa! Aaii!"

(Okay, did not mean to scream like a baby iguana.)

I scrambled up as everyone rushed forward to help.

"I'm okay. I'm okay," I said quickly. (That is, if you didn't count my pride.) Were my cheeks as red as they felt?

I saw Dad out of the corner of my eye. Was he

stifling a laugh?

"You sure?" Carolina asked, as the girls all cooed with concern like I was some kind of injured kitten. I just wanted this little scene to be over.

Then Cassie ruffled my hair again! "Finn's tough," she said brightly. Okay, two hair ruffles: over the line.

Carolina smiled and winked at me. "Well nice to officially meet you Finn. See you guys."

I kind of pointed at her and, before thinking about what I was doing, gave a wink back. But it looked more like a nervous eye twitch. (What was I thinking?!)

And she was off. Hopefully she didn't notice.

I gave Cassie a look that could have shot daggers, which she obviously didn't notice, because she got right back on track with the BMI issue.

"Okay, so, yeah your BMI is 18 and a half. So that's great."

Dad handed her a chart. It looked like a big graph.

"See Finn," she said, running her finger along the paper. "We look at your gender. So, you're a guy."

"Very observant of you Cassie," I joked. (Okay, now my usual sense of humor was back.) Cassie gave me her fake laugh.

"So we use the chart for guys. We look at your age, and your BMI number. And that tells us if you're at a healthy weight."

I watched as she connected the row with my age to the column with my BMI number on the chart.

"It's right there in the middle of the healthy range on the chart," she continued. "You're pretty lean, but you are an active guy, and your metabolism is probably super high," Cassie informed me. "Pretty awesome huh?"

"High metabolism," I echoed. "Should I get that checked?"

This seemed to amuse everyone.

"Your metabolism is like your body's engine and how much it runs," Cassie explained. "Finn, you're on the go all the time, so your muscles are working, your blood's pumping, and all that. If you weren't active, and if you were just laying around all the time and moving really slowly, you'd have a lower metabolism. Your engine wouldn't be running as much."

I think my eyes were still freakishly wide from the load of information, but I said, "Thanks Cassie. Thanks a lot. I really appreciate it."

"No problem," she announced. "I have some good info on healthy weight if you want it."

"Um, okay yeah," I responded, coming out of my math induced stupor. "Are you around this weekend?"

"Sure am. Just text me," she directed. Cassie smiled at me then at her teammates, looking pleased with herself.

Dad, who was now sitting at his desk, chimed in, "Nice job Cass."

Then to me, "Did you know that Cassie just got accepted to the exercise science program at University of North Carolina?" Dad was beaming.

The girls patted her on the back and Cassie looked pumped. "I want to be an exercise physiologist," she nodded to me. "I'm going to work with athletes."

"Wow," I said to Cassie, impressed. "Cool. Congratulations."

"Thanks Finn," Cassie returned, extending her fist to me. I bumped it with mine. "See you Coach," she breezed and the girls exited with waves.

"Thanks Coach. Great practice," Cassie added, and her teammates/backup singers added "Thanks Coach".

Was it just me, or were they all in harmony?

CHAPTER 9

After I snapped out of my math-induced fog, I looked over at Dad. I must have looked stunned, because he laughed and asked, "You want to see an easier way?"

"Heck yeah," I responded. He motioned me toward his computer, and I sat down in the chair next to his.

As I sat down, he stopped and looked at me, a grin threatening to show. "Smooth move on that backward tumble of yours. You sure you didn't hurt anything?"

"Uh Dad, I think the term 'smooth move' is from the 1900's," I countered. "And I'm fine."

He chuckled as he woke up his computer and typed in his password. He turned to me. "So what's this for?" he asked. "Health assignment?"

I shook my head. "Can you keep this on the down low? It's kind of embarrassing," I started.

Dad rotated his chair and faced me directly. He leaned in.

"Son, there's nothing you can't talk to me

about. In fact, you're getting to that age where we really need to have more open communication."

I popped both my hands up in front of me, like I was about to fend off a bear, backtracking.

"For Charlie. It's kind of embarrassing for *Charlie.* Yeah, no, I'm good. Nothing embarrassing of *any* nature on my end."

Dad looked a little wounded. So I blathered on. "But if there was anything, I'd let you know in a second."

Dad straightened up. "Oh good."

I snapped my fingers and pointed at him. "You da man!" I added. (Okay, stop now Finn!)

Was Dad stifling a smile again? Somehow I was being a comedian today without meaning to. Dad re-focused and typed in a website address.

Moving on, I told him about Charlie's situation. "In a nutshell, Charlie's mom took him to see Davis, and he said Charlie's BMI is too high. I mean, he is a little chunky. So now his mom is threatening to take him to that 'ickly' program.

"I C L I," interrupted Dad, trying to keep a straight face. "I Can Lose It?"

"Yeah," I continued. "She's freaking out. And now he's freaking out, so he wanted me to help him. I figured, first thing I'd better do is learn about BMI. I had no idea what it was before this morning."

Dad nodded. "Ah. So that's why Charlie sounded like a chipmunk on Red Bull this morning. Poor guy."

I nodded. "I know," I concurred. "So we just have to figure out a way to get him out of it."

"I know a way," Dad said. "It's called eat less, move more."

"Ooh Dad. Harsh," I countered. "Seriously, I think he's looking for an easier way. Besides, Charlie doesn't eat that much".

"According to who," Dad asked, with eyebrows raised.

"Well, according to him I guess," I answered.

"Did you see him gorging on the triple meat pizza at the school's Italian night? I thought your mom was going to throw up!"

I laughed. "Oh yeah," I remembered.

"So many people underestimate what they eat, Finn, and they always overestimate how healthy they're eating."

I nodded.

"We all have times when we pig out, or when we don't eat as much or keep as active. But Charlie eats a lot and moves very little on a day to day basis," he followed.

Really? Maybe Dad had a point. I guess.

"But that's something to check out later," Dad advised.

I jotted that down in my journal:

EATING and ACTIVITY HABITS OF THE CHARLIE.

This was looking like a science project, with Charlie as my little orangutan.

We looked at the screen. "Okay, so you know what BMI is then?" Dad tested.

"Yeah, it's a way of seeing how much you

weigh compared to your height, to see if it's healthy," I rhymed off. "And it involves an insane equation."

Dad nodded. "Yes. Well, the equation's not that crazy." He stopped and tried to stifle a laugh.

"What?" (Of course I knew what he was trying not to laugh about.)

"You sure you didn't hurt yourself when you fell? Backwards?" He snickered despite himself.

I shook my head, giving him my unimpressed look.

"Pride?"

"Dad!"

"Sorry Finn," he said, focusing again. "Anyway, BMI is just one technique for assessing someone's weight-related health risks. It's not perfect but it's a good indicator and it's quick and non-invasive."

"Non-invasive," I repeated, questioning.

"Non-invasive just means that you don't have to really even touch someone to get the test result," Dad said. "So they don't feel uncomfortable or embarrassed."

"Okay," I nodded.

"Anyway, it's being used more and more because overweight and obesity has become such a problem these days, particularly in kids and teenagers," Dad pointed out.

He gestured to the screen. "Here's a BMI chart for adults. The charts are different for younger folks because you're still growing and developing. So they have a chart that also takes age and gender into consideration. Girls tend to grow at different rates than guys. That's why a lot of the girls in your class are taller than you right now."

I nodded. Yeah, some of the girls in my class had gotten super tall.

"The youth charts use percentiles," Dad continued. "So you're compared to other kids at your age and gender."

"Kids?"

"Dude, someday you're going to be happy to be called a kid," Dad fake-lectured. (Mental note: Must get Dad to stop trying to sound hip by using the term 'dude'.)

"Well, now that I'm thirteen," I started, clearing my throat, "I'm not officially a kid. Just saying."

"Okay, so you're compared to other teenagers," Dad clarified, putting his hands up and doing the bunny ear air quotation marks.

"Cool."

"So," Dad continued, "Cassie said your BMI was around 18. That's normal. Good. You're an active guy and you're naturally lean. No problem. There's a whole range of what's considered healthy. If you had a bit more body fat, that would still be fine. We all need fat."

"Ugh, really?" I made a face.

"Yeah, big time," Dad said matter-of-factly. "Fat does a lot of things for us. It protects our organs," he led off.

I made a face, halfway between surprised and grossed out.

Dad stopped and looked at me. "What?"

"That's kind of gross Dad," I stated. "So, like,

without fat, our organs would just be banging against each other and getting all bruised up?"

Dad shook his head. "It's not like that Finn. But think of fat like a soft protective little blanket."

"Aww."

"Anyway," Dad kept on truckin'. "It also acts as insulation."

I interrupted. "What are we, a bunch of polar bears?"

"Cute," he continued, semi-ignoring my quips. "Some of the vitamins we need are fat-soluble, which means they need fat for us to absorb and use them."

Dad paused, waiting for another smart remark. I had nothing.

"And, we use fat for energy, especially if you're doing something like a hike, paddle, swim, jog, or a bike ride," he finished. "You know, aerobic exercise."

I responded with a very academic sounding, "Huh".

Dad sat back and nodded. "Yep." (Equally academic sounding.)

Dad reached under his computer and grabbed a couple of bananas. (He has food stashed everywhere!) He offered one to me. As I was peeling, I got it.

"So when you hear people talking about fat burning exercise, that's what they're talking about!" I waved the banana at Dad.

"Bingo," he said, catching the top of the banana as it snapped off and flew toward him. (Never use a banana as a pointer.) He ate it.

"I never used to really think about that concept," I finished as I ate the rest of the banana.

"The big issue is when you have way too much fat, too much extra, and you get overweight. Or if you're in a category of being way overweight, and that's considered obese. And more people these days are in those overweight ranges.

I was starting to feel a little concerned for Charlie's well being.

"The kicker is that more and more kids are showing up in the overweight categories," Dad concluded. "So that's probably why Davis focused on that with him. Having a high BMI could cause some health problems for Charlie," Dad added.

Okay, now I was a lot concerned.

Dad turned to look at me. "Did Davis get a chance to talk to him about it?"

"Nope," I answered. "Charlie said his mom rushed him out of there super fast. He said she seemed really embarrassed."

Dad nodded and leaned back. "That makes more sense."

I raised my eyebrows.

Off my look, Dad continued. "I can't see Davis just saying Charlie's overweight without talking to him."

I had to agree there. Davis is a pretty sensitive guy.

I stretched and blinked a few times. "Okay, that's enough new math for one afternoon."

Dad leaned forward again. "Oh yeah, there's

an easier way," he said, tapping a few keys.

A website popped up on the screen. Dad pointed at it.

"This is a BMI calculator," he instructed. "You just fill in your height, weight, gender and age, and poof, it figures out your BMI."

"Cool," I said, impressed.

"Well, it's cool if you know how to use the information," he lectured. "And if you enter everything correctly."

I nodded. (I'm the king of checking my work, so no worries there.)

"I'm going to go over and get Charlie's height and weight and see what his BMI is," I mentioned casually.

Yep, Finn Tilley on the job as a fitness and lifestyle coach.

"I wouldn't do that Finn," Dad said, stopping me in my tracks.

"Why not?" I squeaked. (I have got to work on keeping the voice down.)

"It's great to be aware of BMI and healthy weight ranges and all that," Dad started. "But labeling someone with a number can do more harm than good sometimes."

"Cassie labeled me with a number," I shot back semi-sarcastically. "You don't see me crying."

Dad laughed and shook his head. "But sometimes, people get caught up in the numbers, whether it's BMI or how many pounds they weigh, or clothes sizes."

I was starting to get antsy with realizing it. Pumping my knee up and down, my chair was vibrating. I started tapping my fingers on Dad's desk.

"What Charlie should concentrate on is striking a balance," he started.

I was hitting a good rhythm with the tapping.

Without looking away from the computer, he splatted his hand down on mine. Pretty gently, but point taken. Obviously the finger tapping was getting annoying.

Dad grinned at me. A new screen flashed up on his computer, interrupting his thought. He pressed a button.

"Check this out Finn," he said, directing me to the screen again. "This guy's BMI is 32, so he's in the 'obese' category."

I looked and saw a guy who looked a little like a grown up version of Charlie, if you left out the mustache. My heart sank into my stomach a little.

Dad clicked onto another picture. "This guy's BMI is also 32, so he's also in the 'obese' category.

Whoa. It was a picture of a body builder. The guy was posing and had muscles bulging on his muscles.

"Wait a second," I started.

"This is the big problem with BMI, Finn," Dad said. "It doesn't distinguish between fat weight and lean body weight, like muscle. This bodybuilder has incredibly low body fat. So BMI wouldn't be a good marker of this guy's healthy weight."

"Cool," I said. "Thanks Dad. This is great."

Dad leaned back in his chair. "My pleasure

buddy. Nice to see you."

That's Dad for you: always Mr. Positive. But when I heard a few basketballs bouncing in the gym, I knew he was on again. Guys varsity practice. He looked at his watch.

"Before you go Finn," Dad said, looking at me thoughtfully. "Quick question. Does Fiona snack much after school?"

Kind of a weird question, and frankly I never pay attention to the eating habits of the animal known as my sister. Especially not these days.

"Uh, not really Dad," I answered. "Not that I notice anyway. She's always either dancing, reading, or hanging out with her friends. Or exercising. She never sits still anymore."

"Hmm," my Dad responded, looking a little troubled.

"And she's kind of grumped up all the time."

"Grumped up?"

"Grumpy," I clarified.

"Oh," he nodded, scratching his chin.

"Yeah," I continued. "I mean, every time I see her eat, she's picking at her food."

Dad nodded. "Okay, thanks Finn."

And I kept going. "I mean, that muffin this morning. She looked like a kitten batting the thing around on her plate. I was going to grab it and shove it in my own mouth."

Dad sighed, then laughed despite himself.

The team captain stuck his head in. "Hey Coach," then spotting me, "Hey Finn!"

"Hey Jayson," Dad said enthusiastically. "How's the knee?"

"Doc Jones said I'm clear to play. No restrictions," Jayson said proudly. Then to me, "You want to shoot around with us before practice Finn?"

I stood up. "As much as I'd like to school you yahoos on the court Jay," I joked, "I've got a crazy Labrador retriever waiting for me at home."

(Last time I forgot about taking Ralph out, he grabbed a pair of my mom's yoga pants and chewed them to shreds. Not good. Needless to say, I didn't want to share that little tidbit of information with Jayson.)

Jayson laughed. "Ralph's a superior dog, man," he drawled. "You treat him right."

Dad got up, caught me in a big playful neck hold, then ruffled the hair on top of my head. (What was it with my hair today? Seriously.)

Luckily, Dad can show affection without being too mushy. He comes from a family of huggers, so I give him some slack. Also lucky that I was going for the messy look in the hair department.

"If you want to shoot for a few minutes Finn, I'm sure Ralph can cross his legs," Dad said, erasing the white board.

Ah, what the heck, I thought. Basketball will never be my main sport, but I do play pick up with the guys now and then. I can hold my own (barely) and believe me, I know how lucky I am to be included. It's fun and I always end up learning something new. The guys are awesome, and I don't think they're being nice just because I'm the coach's son. They're not 'suck up' kind of guys.

I nodded. "Okay, cool," I said to Jayson. "As

long as you don't mind me kicking your ass-"

"Ahem."

I looked at Dad who did the menacing throat clear again. Oops. I don't know what's worse to Dad: His kid saying 'the-other-word-for-butt', or showing false bravado? (Dad's a real 'don't talk about it, just get out there and do it' kind of guy.)

Jayson was looking around the office, trying to stifle a laugh.

"I mean, yeah, sorry Jay. Let's jam," I corrected myself. (Let's jam?? Where'd I get that line?)

I breezed out in front of Jayson. Dad grabbed his whistle and clipboard. He patted Jayson on the shoulder. "Jay, Coach Langford is away today." (That's the assistant coach.) "Can you start the warm up?" he asked.

That meant grabbing the stereo, blasting some pump-up music, and getting the guys moving. They always do that for warm-up. Dad says it gets everyone loosened up and ready to play. I believe it. I love listening to music when we're warming up for tennis practice.

"Sure thing Coach," Jayson pumped back.

I can tell that Jayson and the rest of the guys respect Dad. He's had the team over for suppers (you don't even want to know how much food these guys go through), and they get advice from him when they're making a big decision. He writes references for them for university. He's also helped a couple of guys out who don't really have a great life at home. Dad makes sure the team is like a family. Pretty cool.

I shot around for a few minutes with the guys.

This is what I like best, just goofing around, seeing what you can do. No pressure.

Everyone was talking, shooting, really chilled out. It's a great atmosphere. The team does seem pretty tight, like they're friends off the court too.

I made a few good shots. A couple of the guys can dunk and they were trying to one-up each other. There were a couple of epic slams. These guys are so talented. And they just love to play.

After about ten minutes, I looked at my watch. Besides Ralph's bladder, the other urgent matter was calling Charlie and getting his height and weight. Charlie would be fine with it. I just wanted to see what we were dealing with.

I grabbed my backpack and sauntered toward Dad, backpack slung over my shoulder. I waved to the guys, still shooting baskets and stretching with the music pumping. As I got near Dad, I gave him a casual wave and pointed toward the door.

"See you in a while buddy," he replied. He grabbed me in a one armed hug and gave me a kiss on the top of the head. So much for a smooth exit.

CHAPTER 10

After I got hauled around the block courtesy of Ralph, I got out my notebook and plunked down in my favorite chair in the den. It's this old corduroy chair-and-a-half so it's extra wide. You can really sprawl out in it. Plus, the arms are wide so you can balance your snack.

Mom was out teaching a class but she had made me a little fruit plate and some yogurt dip. Usually I fend for myself in the 'after school snack' department, so I made a mental note to thank her.

Ralph tried to shimmy his way up on the chair beside me. I realized I had put a doggie treat in my pocket for him, so I gave it a little toss. Perfect catch! (Ralph has excellent mouth-eye coordination.)

Ralph was happy, and pretty disinterested in my fruit plate, so he settled on the floor by my chair – within patting distance of me.

Mm, the fruit would be good for a start. I don't know if it was all the math, but I was starving. Maybe I'd make a shake after.

I didn't know where Fiona was, but she was probably at dance. That girl does so many different kinds of dancing, it's crazy, but ballet is her main gig.

I wondered why Dad had asked about her snacks. It's not like she doesn't have any variety. Mom has hauled us both to the grocery store to pick out healthy stuff that we'll actually eat. (Somehow, on the first trip, she didn't agree that the Frosted Rainbow Fruity-O's I picked out were healthy. Hmm.)

I surfed the channels for a few minutes. We're not supposed to watch a lot of t.v. but the folks say it's okay to pop it on for a few minutes if it's educational. (They haven't set a screen time limit like a lot of my friends' parents, as long as we don't "abuse the t.v., computer, phones, etc.")

This time of day there wasn't a lot on. I flicked through a bunch of talk shows. I paused at one. The First Lady was on, talking about getting kids moving. (That's one of her big mandates.) She is pretty cool. And wow, she's got pipes! You have to admire that. I wonder if she ever takes President Obama on in hoops. Yikes, they were talking about how our generation is something like the most inactive ever. Really?

And, commercial break.

I popped on ESPN. That's educational. Sort of?! I hit the mute button, and dialed Charlie's number.

As usual, Josie answered. She's Charlie's maid, or housekeeper, or whatever you want to call it. (They also have a cook, a gardener, and a butler/

driver! Charlie used to have a nanny, but when he turned thirteen, she went back to England. She was nice but pretty strict.)

"Good afternoon. Bienenstock residence," Josie chimed in a sophisticated voice.

"Hey Josie, it's Finn," I answered. "How are you today?"

"Hi Finn, well I'm good thanks," Josie returned, in a warm tone. Josie likes me, I think mainly because I'm polite and take a minute to ask how she's doing. I think she's really cool too.

"Would you like to speak to Charlie," she continued.

"Yeah, please," I said, waiting for it.

I heard her call out, "Master Charlie, Master Finn is on the telephone for you." (That always cracks me up!)

There was a pause, then I heard Charlie says thanks and pick up another line.

"Hell-ooh Mah-stah Chahhhles," I boomed in my best (yet still crappy) British accent.

"Hey mate," Charlie responded flatly. Not only has he heard me say that line about a thousand times, he was still bummed out.

I felt for the poor guy, so I got down to business. "Hey, I need your height and weight," I said. "Do you know it?"

Again, I detected a whimper. "I can't remember what it is. I was so caught off guard at the doctor's office."

"Can you get it?" I asked.

"Yeah, I suppose. Uh," he tapered off. He sounded nervous all of a sudden.

I remembered what Dad had just said about not labeling Charlie with a number. But I just wanted to get an idea. He'd be cool with it.

I popped a piece of melon in my mouth. "Want me to come over with a tape measure?" I asked, knowing the answer.

Charlie sighed. "Well, yes I suppose so."

"I mean, Doc Jones could have made a mistake."

"Alright then," he sighed. "Would you?"

I licked the rest of the dip out of the bowl and got up.

After I put my dishes in the sink, I pulled open the junk drawer in the kitchen. It's not really filled with junk. It's just messy. But somehow you can always find what you need in it. I rummaged around and found a tape measure. See what I mean?

I left a note for Mom and grabbed my notebook before popping out the back door.

Charlie's house is approximately a minute and a half from mine, if you take the shortcut.

See, he lives on 'Mansion Alley', as everyone calls it.

Our place is small and kind of old, but it's in the historical section of town, which is next to the super rich section. Plus, our house is pretty homey, with lots of comfy furniture, pottery, and pictures. It's kind of crowded but everyone feels welcome and pretty relaxed when they come in, so that's cool.

Mom and Dad inherited our place from Mom's great aunt, who never had any kids, but was close to Mom. So I guess it pays to be nice to your old relatives.

I crossed my backyard, hopped the fence, jogged down a small path, and voila, I was in Charlie's backyard (if you want to call it that). Charlie's folks call his yard 'the grounds'.

I jogged past the tennis court, then by the pool and pool house (which, funny enough, has a pool table), and slowed to a walk as I got to the kitchen entrance.

I knocked and Alice, their chef, answered the door. As expected, she was baking cookies. Yes! It was chocolate chip day.

As Alice opened the door, the aroma wafted toward me, surrounding me like a warm embrace...

(Sorry! Just practicing for my English essay. But man it smelled good!)

"Your timing is impeccable Finn," she laughed.

"Hi Alice," I said sweetly, walking in. "Wow, it smells awesome in here. As usual." (In case you're wondering: Yes, of course I was sucking up!)

Charlie's kitchen is approximately the size of some college apartments. It's huge! Seriously, it's like walking into a restaurant kitchen, all humongous silver appliances, and tons of space to move around. There are two work islands and two large wooden tables with big vases of flowers on them (one for the family, one for the staff), plus a bunch of sinks and all that. It's so big, we ride our scooters here sometimes, not that it goes over real well.

Alice popped a few cookies off a cooling rack, put them on a plate, and set them down on the table. "Would you like some Finn?" She smiled, knowing the answer was an absolute yes. I grabbed one.

"Thanks a lot," I gushed.

These weren't just any chocolate chip cookies. For one thing, they were huge. The other thing is that they have three kinds of chocolate: milk, dark, and white. Wow.

Charlie sauntered in, still obviously in a funk. I glanced at his arms and his mid-section, which both looked kind of soft and doughy. Not a muscle in sight. They were hiding in there somewhere. (Thinking back to seeing Mrs. Obama and her pipes on that talk show, she could definitely take Charlie in an arm wrestle.)

Unfortunately, I didn't think Charlie had the same problem as the bodybuilder.

"Hey mate." (I like how they say "Hey pal" in England.)

He sat down, grabbed a cookie, and started shoving it in his mouth, not unlike a certain blue monster I remember from my Sesame Street days. (Although, didn't I hear the Cookie Monster is now into veggies too? Maybe he has a fitness and lifestyle coach.)

Charlie seemed to brighten up a little.

"Hey, I just spoke to Tom and Xavier and they're in for tomorrow night too," he told me.

We were all sleeping over at Charlie's tomorrow night.

"Awesome," I pumped back. "It'll be a blast!"

After he demolished the cookie, he reached for another. "Thank you Alice," he said between chomps. I nodded and managed a muffled "so good", with a melted chocolate-filled mouth.

"You're welcome guys." She smiled at us and busied herself in another part of the kitchen.

I slapped the tape measure on the table as I finished my cookie.

"Let's do this," I commanded.

Charlie was still in major cookie mode, now starting a third. "Don't you want another one?" he asked.

I put up my hand. "Those are triple size cookies man," I shot back. I opened my notebook and made a note in the eating habits section:

Subject is able to eat 3 triple size cookies without barfing.

"I'm a growing lad," Charlie protested, sounding stressed. "I have to eat."

"You don't have to eat the leg off the table," I shot back.

He dropped the last (tiny) morsel of his cookie with this big, melodramatic sigh.

"Well you might as well eat the last chocolate chip if it means that much to you."

"Ha ha," Charlie shot back. But he picked up that morsel and popped it in his mouth.

When I slapped my head and shook it, he went on rationalizing. "It was just sitting there all lonely on the plate. I don't want to waste food."

"Dude. Just so we're on the same page here," I lectured, "chocolate chips don't have feelings!"

Charlie laughed. "Blimey, that would make a

great improv for my next drama class."

He looked at me, serious again. "I know, I'm just bummed up and these make me happy. It's only a few cookies."

"Bummed out," I corrected. (Sometimes Charlie forgets the nuances of American sayings.) "Bummed up sounds like you're constipated."

He laughed again, despite himself.

I scribbled quickly:

Cookies are big mood booster.

I was starting to realize the problem here. Obviously Charlie was in denial. I got up. "Where's your scale?"

Charlie sighed this big melodramatic, sad-puppy-dog kind of sigh.

I looked around the room, then looked Charlie right in the eye. I asked, "Does this look like 'American Idol' to you?"

Charlie raised one eyebrow. "No," he started.

"Nobody's judging you man," I followed. "Let's go."

(By the way, I have an embarrassing yet humbling story about judging people. I'll tell you about it in my notebook, at the end.)

Charlie rose slowly, grunting as he stood up. "Alright, fine. Come on," he muttered.

I followed him as we headed to another wing. (I told you his house is huge.) "Where's Beatrice?" I asked.

By the way, we never actually call Charlie's mom 'Beatrice' in front of her. She and Charlie's dad are the only parents we actually call by their surnames. When I see her, it's all 'Hello Mrs. Bienenstock, how are you Mrs. Bienenstock, lovely day we're having Mrs. Bienenstock', that sort of thing.

"I don't know," Charlie muttered again as we walked along. "Out at some charity meeting I think. Dad's in London for another few days."

(Charlie's dad is president of some huge global company, so when he flies it's usually on the corporate jet! Talk about lifestyles of the rich and famous. And the Bienenstocks!)

"I heard her talking to Dad on the phone about me," Charlie complained. "She said if ICLI doesn't work, perhaps a camp."

"Hey, camp's fun," I replied optimistically. "Maybe I could go for a week too," I started.

"Fat camp," he stated.

Oh.

"Charlie, I don't think they call it that," I soothed. "And anyway, it won't get to that."

Once we got to the other wing, we went upstairs to his main bathroom. He stepped on the scale.

I looked at the reading: 140

A hundred and forty pounds! Whoa!

Charlie stepped off. "Got a ruler?" I asked. We walked into his room and he grabbed a ruler off his desk.

I got Charlie to stand against the wall, and held the ruler straight across the top of his noggin. While he held the spot with his finger, I measured. Charlie had gotten a little quiet after stepping off the scale.

"Let's see," I read, looking at the measure. "Five foot four."

Hmm, Charlie was only a little taller than me. He always seems way taller.

Charlie looked at me. "What do you think?"

I cocked my head to the side. "Dad showed me how to figure this out. Here, I'll show you the website," I said, heading to Charlie's homework room.

Charlie's homework room is basically an office, but just for him. His mom doesn't want a computer in his room. Meanwhile, I get to compete for our computer at the kitchen desk nook. Between Mom and her recipes, and Fiona's Harry Stiles stalking, it's no picnic.

There was a script on the desk. I picked it up.

"Hey, what're you working on?"

Charlie brightened up, as he always does when he's talking or thinking about acting.

"It's for my drama class," he said with a little more energy. "We're focusing on balance when you're on the stage."

"Like, what do you mean? Keeping your balance?" I stood on one foot and grinned.

Charlie smiled, totally engaged. "Balance in terms of how you project your voice, when you're speaking or singing. It depends on the mood of the scene and what not. So the audience can hear you well, but you don't sound like you're shouting."

"Oh, yeah. Cool."

"Maybe you could run some lines with me later," Charlie offered.

(I have to tell you, I've run lines with Charlie before. It just means I read the lines of other characters so he can practice how his character speaks when he's in a play. It's actually really fun to get into different characters. Charlie's really good at totally immersing himself in how a character speaks. He does a bang up American accent when he has to. And even a Canadian one, which I never thought we had.)

I put the script down. "Yeah, great. Whenever you want. But let's finish this."

We turned on Charlie's computer and I found the website Dad showed me for kids and teenagers.

Before I entered his numbers, I showed him the chart with the health classifications. They also had some cool info about BMI. Sort of like how it affects your health. Charlie wiped a crumb off his cheek distractedly as he looked at some of the nasty stuff associated with being way too heavy. Stuff like risk of heart disease when you get older, stress on your joints, and higher chance of diabetes. Some of the stuff Ms. Bowden had talked about.

You know how it is: When you're thirteen, you don't really think about heart disease or any of that stuff a whole lot. That's for when you're older. Saying that, I now get why Charlie complains that his knees are always sore.

I think what freaked Charlie out is that the list of bad health problems is so long.

They don't list 'bruised pride' on there, but it should definitely be on the list.

I entered the numbers and got 24.8, so really just about **25**. I looked at the percentiles. Whoa, **25: Overweight**. Charlie's face fell. So did my jaw.

I patted him on the shoulder. "So this is our starting point," I began.

I looked at Charlie. He was, for the first time, speechless. And he was kind of pale. He looked really defeated.

The funny thing is, Charlie knew there was a problem, because he hasn't been feeling all that great. He's been really low energy and run down. That's probably why Beatrice took him to see Davis in the first place. But when you see something specific on paper, like this, it really brings it home.

Dad was right, I shouldn't have started with defining his weight with a BMI number and category.

He stared at me and shook his head.

So I followed with a very eloquent: "What?"

"This is terrible mate," he stuttered. He was about to continue when I stopped him.

"Hold up Charlie," I boomed. (I had to get his attention before his voice went to female chipmunk range.) "This number doesn't define you. This number isn't who you are. Does this number stand for Charlie Bienenstock, the coolest best friend around, awesome actor, and all around warm and fuzzy guy who everyone loves? Heck no!"

(Man, I should coach competitive sports some day!)

I continued. "This is your starting point. Now

you know you should deal with this. That's our first step. Doing it while avoiding ICLI is our second step."

Charlie looked down at his feet. I felt bad.

"Okay then," I continued to boom. "We're gonna get it done!"

Charlie forced a tense smile and nodded as I got up. The question was, what we were going to do next.

CHAPTER 11

I didn't hang out for long after that. Once I talked Charlie down, literally – his voice went up to opera/screech level – I told him I was going to get my stuff together and come up with a plan.

Anyway, it was Friday night. That's Movie Night at my place. I'd see Charlie in about an hour and a half.

I scooted home. Seriously, I had left my scooter at Charlie's house the other day, so I hopped on and took the longer way. I was really looking forward to turning my brain off with a movie.

I parked my scooter around back and came in through the kitchen.

Mom was at the counter and some old (or as Mom calls it, 'classic') 1980's dance music was playing.

Mom can't sit still when her tunes are on, and I'll admit she's actually got some moves.

That is except for what we like to call the 'snap and clap', (snapping her fingers and clapping her hands at various intervals) that was obviously popular way back when.

When she throws in an "Ow!" it's really funny.

Mom saw me and called out her usual "Hey buddy". (I had finally trained her out of 'Honey Bun').

I took my sneakers off and approached. She turned and gave me a kiss on the head. "Hey Mom," I returned.

"Thanks for the note," she said. "Are Charlie and Chris coming over tonight?" I nodded.

She was still kind of dancing in place. The fact that this woman actually calms down enough to sit on a mat, let alone teach an entire yoga class – daily! – that irony does not escape me.

She held up her hands like a surgeon preparing to operate, and they looked like they were coated in Corn Flakes. That's because they were.

"I'm making chicken fingers for dinner," she told me. "Did you get your snack?" She washed her hands and put the chicken fingers in the oven.

I turned down the iPod. "Yeah, thanks," I said appreciatively. "That dip was great!"

"It's just yogurt and a little honey." Hmm, impressively simple.

I nodded and sat down at the table.

"Where's Ralph?" I was surprised he wasn't here, fawning all over me.

"He was here a few minutes ago, mooching," Mom laughed. "I gave him a little chewy bone."

Ralph, now hearing my voice instead of Madonna's, came running. He had the little rawhide stick, so it looked like he had a cigar in his mouth. He dropped it when he saw me. (That's love.)

"There you are Ralphie," I exclaimed as he tried to coat me with major dog slobber. I got down on the floor with him. I scratched his back, near his hips. He loves that. He gets this look on his face like, 'you are the best person in the whole universe'.

When I got up in the chair again, he put his chin on my lap and looked at me with that 'I love you man' expression again. Then he picked up his chewy stick and moseyed around, wagging his tail.

Mom actually stopped moving for a minute. "Want something to nibble before dinner?"

I rubbed my stomach. "Oh, no thanks," I shook my head. "I had one of Alice's cookies. They are huge! I still feel full."

Mom went to the sink as I got up to feed Ralph. "How is Charlie," she half-asked, half-stated. She turned around and looked at me, her head cocked to the side a little. "He seemed a little nervous this morning."

I scooped Ralphie's kibble into his bowl and leaned against the counter while he wolfed down his food.

"He's all upset because he went to see Davis, and Davis said his BMI is too high, and his mom is threatening to take him to Icky," I started.

"ICLI," Mom corrected, stifling a laugh.

"So he asked me to help him check into BMI and it's pretty bad," I continued. Mom nodded as I spoke. "I mean, I didn't realize how much your weight affects your health. Charlie's a walking time bomb!"

Mom chuckled. "Okay Mr. Dramatic, what is his BMI?"

"Twenty five," I shot back casually.

"Holy crap!" Mom shouted. "And the boy's thirteen?!"

"And a quarter," I corrected her.

Just then, Dad and Fiona walked in. Fiona was still in her dance clothes (minus the tutu). Dad called his usual "Hey guys" and kissed Mom.

Fiona, who can smell drama a mile away, stopped and put both hands in front of her. "What's up," she asked in an urgent tone.

"Nothing, Drama Queen," I said. "It's between Mom and me."

Mom looked at Dad. "John, Charlie's BMI is twenty five!"

So much for confidentiality.

Dad looked at me. "Seriously?"

I nodded.

"Hold it, I didn't think you were going to get his specific BMI," Dad said. "You were just going to talk to him about getting a little more active and paying more attention to what he's eating."

"I thought he could take it," I shrugged.

Dad cocked his head to the side a la Ralph and gave me his 'why didn't you listen to me' look.

"Maybe this will jolt him into action," I followed hopefully.

Mom and Dad both looked at me with raised eyebrows.

Mom turned down the music a little more. "Is he going to see Davis again?"

"He didn't mention it," I answered.

Dad seemed lost in thought. "And you're sure you entered his height and weight the right way," Dad continued. I nodded again.

Fiona was looking wildly back and forth between us. "What? What's going on? Is Charlie sick?" she stuttered.

Then she added, out of the blue, "Is Tom coming over?" (Fiona has recently developed a big crush on Tom. I usually ignore it, lest I feel like hurling. Luckliy, he's pretty laid back about it.)

I cocked my head at her, again a la Ralph. (He really rubs off on us!)

"I mean," she continued.

"Listen Fifi, MY friend Tom is not coming over tonight. And what we're talking about, it's a little personal," I reprimanded her.

She scrunched up her nose and widened her eyes at me like some sort of pig/ferret mix. "Don't call me Fifi!"

I smiled sweetly at her. "Come on Fifi, it's just my pet name for you."

"Do I look like a poodle to you?!"

I opened my mouth to answer-

"Finn!" Mom looked down her nose at me. "Fifi, er uh Fiona is just concerned. We all love Charlie."

Fiona looked at Mom and Dad with her fake angelic look and nodded, which they somehow bought. (Barf.)

"So what's the deal?" she pressed. "Is it embarrassing? Is he coming over tonight? Should I act like everything's normal?"

"Yes yes," I said, exasperated.

"Yes what?" Fiona followed, a little too excited. "Embarrassing?"

Luckily Mom interrupted her little interrogation.

"Are you hungry?" Mom asked Fiona this question as if she was a lawyer in a courtroom, and Fiona was the defendant. Mom put her hand on Fiona's arm.

Fiona shook her head. Mom looked at Dad with super wide eyes (like a Muppet), then at Fiona, as if Fiona had done something wrong.

"What did you have to eat after school and before dance?" Dad asked her.

Fiona shrugged her shoulders.

"I'd like you to have a little snack," Mom prodded Fiona.

"I'm not hungry, seriously," Fiona protested.

I was looking back and forth at these guys. What was the deal with the snack drama?

"Just have a carrot stick and make the folks happy," I joked.

Mom picked up a hoodie. "Come on up and change Fi," she said. "I've got to put away some laundry. And I want to have a little chit chat."

Ooh, whenever Mom uses the term 'chit chat', it usually means you're in trouble.

They both left the kitchen, Fiona rolling her eyes.

I looked at Dad. "So what do you think?"

"I think her ballet teacher is telling her to lose weight," Dad said grimly. He looked like he was kind of upset.

What the heck? Here I was dealing with too

much weight. I never thought too little weight was a problem. (I was also surprised because Fiona is not exactly the size of a linebacker to start with, if you get my drift. I mean, how much weight can she lose?)

"Oh, uh. I meant about Charlie," I mumbled. "But wow, why would her teacher ask her to lose weight when she's already tiny?"

Dad looked like he had a thundercloud over his head. He sighed. "I don't know."

"Want me to say something to Fiona?"

Dad snapped out of it. "Thanks Finn but we'll deal with it for now."

"Okay, well, I'll just figure out how to help out Charlie."

He went to the fridge and got out the milk, motioning to me. I said yes with a thumb's up. Dad poured a glass of milk for each of us, came over with them, and we both took a swig.

"Well, Finn, it's obvious Charlie has to lose weight. He'll feel way better if he does. What's the big issue for him?"

That's what I like about Dad. He gets right to the heart of things.

I patted Ralph. "He doesn't want to be dragged to ICLI."

Dad shrugged. "ICLI helps a lot of people. But I can understand how he wouldn't want to go at his age. Honestly Finn, it's a simple deal. Charlie just has to burn more calories than he's taking in."

I must have looked blank because Dad sat down and launched into his lecture voice.

"Do you know what a calorie actually is,

Finn?" he asked.

"Yeah, of course," I returned. "It's the stuff in food that makes you get fat."

"Partly right," said Dad. "Calories are a measure of energy. So we know how many calories are in different types of food. And we know how many calories you burn when you do different activities."

I looked at Dad blankly.

"And when you burn calories, it creates heat," he continued gamely.

"Heat?" Okay, now I was confused.

"Like I say, it's a unit of energy." Dad shifted. "What do you do when you play a hard game of tennis?

I shrugged. "Win?"

Dad laughed. "I like that, Killer." He paused. "But you do another thing. You sweat, right? It's the same when you run or do any other exercise. When you exercise, you get hot. Your body burns calories as fuel and creates heat as a result. The more intense the exercise, the more calories burned, the more heat. So if you play tennis hard, you're going to get hot. If you go for a walk, you're still burning calories and creating heat. It's just not necessarily as noticeable."

…And the proverbial lightbulb just switched on over my head. "Ah," I nodded.

"So Charlie is taking in lots of energy in calories," Dad continued. "But he's not burning it, not using it. So the calories get converted to stored energy."

Oh, so that's good," I said, upbeat. "He should

have lots of extra energy."

"The energy is stored as fat," Dad added.

"Oh, so that's bad," I said, back to downbeat.

"So, that's why he has to burn more calories than he eats, if he wants to lose weight. He has to lose some fat."

I raised my eyebrows. "That could be tough. He ate three of Alice's giant chocolate chip cookies a little while ago. As a light snack."

"Wow," Dad muttered. "That's a brutal combination. He's eating high fat, high calorie foods, with not a lot of nutrition. And he's not moving a lot."

I gave Dad an incredulous look. "He moves."

"Not much Finn," Dad said seriously. "He doesn't do any sports. And that's fine. You don't need to do an organized sport to be fit. But he's not active in general. He doesn't have balance between what he eats and what he burns off. He gets lots of rides to places, and you've said he spends a lot of time sitting in front of his tv and his Xbox."

"Plus his Wii, his computer, his iPad, his iPhone," I added. (Wow, that is a lot of screen time.)

Dad thought for a moment. "And that's the problem with kids today."

My eyebrows went up like two surprised caterpillars.

"Did I just sound like Gramps?" he asked, knowing the answer.

I gave the only appropriate response. "Yep."

"You should ask him sometime what it was like when he was a kid," Dad advised.

RING! It was the phone. One glance at caller

ID and I had to laugh. It was Gramps. He has an uncanny ability to call at exactly the right time.

"Mind if I grab it," I said as I grabbed it anyway.

Dad gave the thumb's up. "I'll talk with him after you." He pointed upstairs and left the room.

I picked up. "Phil's Pizza!"

Without missing a beat, and completely on fire: "Hey there young whippersnapper! I'll have a large veggie!" Gramps said, laughing. "How are you big guy?"

(Now you understand where my dad gets it from.)

"I'm awesome," I shot back. For an old guy, Gramps has the ability to pump you up within ten seconds of talking to him. "How are you?"

"Fantastic, my boy," he returned. "Just played two sets of tennis and I feel like a million bucks! How's your tennis going? You going to be beating the pros soon or what?"

"Yeah, soon Gramps, but they're all too scared to play me," I joked.

Then, changing tone, and realizing this could open up a whole can of worms, "I have a question for you."

"Hit me."

"Well, Dad and I were talking about how active kids are these days, and he said you had to do more physical activity back in the olden days."

Gramps laughed. "Oh yes Finn. Everyone had chores. I had to chop wood for our woodstove. That was our only source of heat. And we all had to tend the garden. And of course there was Trixie," he said, softening his tone. "She kept me real busy."

Okay, just to fill you in: Trixie was Gramps' cow. And beloved pet. I had only heard of her about five hundred times.

"Did I ever tell you how I had to walk her to the pasture at six a.m. after milking her? Then walk her back at suppertime?"

"Yeah, I think so," I answered. Like I say, five hundred times. (This was when I wished we had a chair by the phone.)

"She was a good cow," Gramps said, sounding wistful.

And, getting back on track.

"So Gramps, what would your typical day be?"

"Well, I'd get up at five in the morning, help my brothers bring some wood in, milk Trixie, walk her the half mile down the road to the pasture so she could graze and be with her cow friends. That was nice for her. Then I'd walk back, clean the barn, have breakfast, walk the mile to school with my brothers and sisters, then walk back after, tend the garden, chop some more wood, shovel snow, or help in the house, depending on the season, then do my homework, bring Trixie back and milk her again, eat, maybe read, or Mama would read to all of us. Otherwise, we'd listen to the radio or tell stories, and then go to bed."

Holy. Smokes.

"Seriously?" I know I sounded a little disbelieving.

"Well, yes," Gramps said matter-of-factly. "That was life. We weren't rich and we lived in the country. If you wanted milk or warmth, you had to make it happen. So it was a very physical lifestyle."

"What about the girls?"

"They did the housework, made bread every day, picked berries in summer, made jams, pickles, and all kinds of other things, mended clothes, and tended the garden also," Gramps informed me. "We all did chores together so it wasn't bad. We didn't have a Stop N Shop around the corner. We made a lot of things ourselves."

"Wow," I said, a little flatly.

"And in our family, the girls could do most things the boys did. My sister Helen could split wood for kindling like nobody's business. She's still got a good set of biceps on her."

"We've got it pretty easy," I mused.

"I mean, we had a lot of fun too," Gramps told me. "We went swimming at the pond in the summer, and skating and sliding in the winter. After our chores were done. And there was a nice sense of accomplishment to chopping a bunch of wood, or harvesting veggies from the garden. Made you feel good, you know?"

Then, sounding wistful again, "And I didn't mind walking Trixie to and from the pasture. I loved that cow."

(I had to say something.) "Gee Gramps, she sounds like she was a really special cow."

I would have laughed at this whole 'reminiscing about your pet cow' scenario, if I weren't so stunned by the amount of work kids had to do back in Gramps' day.

"She sure was. And Finn, one last thing. We were lucky," Gramps followed. "A couple of my friends had to drop out of school as teenagers to help support their families."

"Seriously?" I said incredulously. "Was that, like, legal?"

Gramps laughed but then sounded kind of serious. "It was just the way it was, Finn."

Again: Wow.

"And Finn, not to sound like an old relic or anything, but kids were really pretty happy in those days. I love my iPad and all," he added. "But there was a sense of camaraderie and pride at getting things done. It was a simple life but it was good."

"Seriously Gramps?"

He laughed. "Remember when you built that tree fort with your dad a couple of years ago?"

"Yeah," I replied, remembering how much fun we had doing it.

"That's what it was like. A sense of accomplishment at the end of each day."

"I never thought of it that way. Well, thanks Gramps," I said sincerely.

"My pleasure kiddo," he replied.

"You want to talk to Dad?"

Then, back to his usual pumped-up-gramps tone, "Oh shoot, I just looked at the time. I've got to run. We're building a new kennel at the SPCA. Give everyone a big hug from me and tell your dad I was just checking in."

"Okay Gramps. Thanks again."

"Anytime Finn," he said, followed by, "And

keep working on that tennis. You don't want your gramps to whup your butt next time we play!"

And, with a laugh, he was gone. I hung up the phone.

Dad walked back in, and looked at me quizzically. "Everything okay with Gramps?"

"Yep. He's on fire as usual," I informed him. "Just checking in."

Dad shook his head, smiling. "I'll call him back later."

He sat on the counter. "What I meant to say before – and this would be a great project – is that we all don't have to do as much physical work as we used to. That's cool, because there's more time for leisure activities and fun. But sometimes having all our conveniences just makes people less active."

"Yeah Dad, I get what you're saying," I nodded. "Especially after talking to Gramps."

Dad nodded. "You know what? If you're worried about Charlie, Davis could give you some advice. We're going for a run tomorrow. He'll probably pop in for some coffee after."

"Davis already told him there was a problem," I said.

Dad got up and started slicing a baguette. "Yeah, but it sounded like his mom freaked out and rushed him out of there before he could learn anything."

(Okay, I've got to tell you, it cracks me up when Dad says stuff like 'freaked out'. I mean, I think he's trying to be cool, and to connect with me, and all that. So I let it go.)

"Yeah," I agreed. "Charlie said she was super embarrassed."

"They should make an appointment to see him again," Dad continued. "He could have given them some great resources if his mom had been open to it."

I smiled and nodded. "Okay, thanks Dad. Actually though, maybe I'll call Davis. Charlie's my friend and all."

Dad winked. "Good idea. Way to take action, Finn."

"In the meantime," I mused, "I'm going to keep an eye on how much Charlie eats tonight."

CHAPTER 12

Dad left the kitchen again to get changed. He actually gets home and dresses up: He changes from sweats at work to jeans at home. That's my kind of job.

I went to the phone and looked up Davis' office number. Since he's also our family doctor and injuries guru, it's listed on our 'important numbers' board.

I dialed, pacing back and forth as it rang. It's not like I was nervous; we just don't have a chair by the phone. Supposedly it's better for us to stand up or move around while we blab. Plus, it keeps Fiona's gossip-fests from going on for over an hour.

Davis is in practice with a few other doctors who do family practice and internal medicine. Davis is the only one who also does sports medicine. If I was ever going to be a doctor, that's what I'd do. I don't know about the whole blood and gore aspect though.

As it is, I'm undecided on my future career

plans. It's funny: You go from knowing what you want to do at age five - firefighter, policeman, cowboy, or in Charlie's case, Academy Award winning actor - to not having a sweet clue. Although, come to think of it, Charlie still wants to be an actor.

"Family practice and sports medicine associates," chirped the voice on the other end of the line. I snapped out of it.

"Hello, may I speak with Dr. Jones," I inquired seriously.

A slight pause.

"Who may I say is calling?" she continued. Did I detect a smile in her tone?

"It's Finn Tilley. I'm a friend of Dr. Jones. Is he with a patient?"

"Yes Mr. Tilley," she said, sort of mock-seriously, in an I'm-talking-to-a-three-year-old voice. "He *is* with a patient at the moment. Would you like to leave him a little message?"

Okay, so she was playing with me here. Give me a break. Yes, I'm a kid. I get it. Just get Davis on the horn.

"That would be great. Again, it's Finn Tilley. The number is 555-4822," I stated coolly. "And who am I speaking with?"

Another pause, and I think I detected a change in tone. "It's Brenda. I'll give him the message."

"Thanks Brenda," I finished, and hung up.

I stood there for a second, and then dialed Chris' number. She answered midway through the first ring.

"Hey Chris, it's Finn," I said. "That was quick."

"Yeah, I'm in the kitchen. I've got to help with dinner. Dad's coming over but he's running late," she responded. "Movie night still on?"

"Yeah, usual time," I said. "Listen, I need your opinion."

"Yeah? Shoot." I heard a clatter of pans in the background. Then, under her breath, "Oh crap."

"You good?" I asked. I could hear more background noise. I had to stifle a laugh.

Chris groaned. "Uh huh. Uh, hold on."

I don't know why Chris's mom lets her even step into the kitchen. (She got her to do the laundry once, but Chris forgot to check pockets and one of her brothers had left a couple of highlighters in his. They all ended up with a bunch of tie-died clothes.) She's a spaz with a capital S.

Chris's mom is a nurse and her dad is a business guy with pretty long hours. Her parents are divorced, but it's a 'friendly divorce'. So Chris and her brothers live with her mom most of the time, but their dad lives nearby, and is still welcome in the house, and they seem to get along pretty well for being split up.

In any case, Chris has to be pretty independent sometimes. Luckily Chris has two older brothers who dote on her. (There's enough space between them that she never got in their hair.) That's also probably the reason Chris is not a frilly girly-girl. My theory is that big brothers tend to toughen you up. (Which makes me wonder what's happened to Fiona lately.)

I'd bet five bucks that one of them is springing for take-out. Again.

I heard muffled voices, then she said, "Really? Oh man, thanks. I owe you one."

She came back on the phone. "I kind of had a little mishap with the noodles so Matt's ordering pizza."

See what I mean?

"Cool. Anyway," I led. "Charlie is having a bit of a problem with his weight. Do you notice what he eats?"

Chris snorted. "Notice? The question is, have you *not* noticed? He eats like a bull!"

Okaaaay. No sitting on the fence on that one.

"Yeah, but lots of people eat a lot at our age," I countered. "I assume he needs to eat that much because of growth."

"He *is* growing. Out," snapped Chris.

"You're sympathetic," I snapped back, half-joking.

"I mean, I don't know," Chris continued. "Xavier can shovel it back. So can I for that matter. But Xav's like a toothpick. And I'm not exactly huge either. Charlie is a really big guy."

"Hmm," I said, thinking out loud. "That's true. Anyway, don't say anything but Beatrice is all freaked out about his weight. Davis told him his BMI is too high."

Chris stopped me. "His what?"

I gave her the ten-second explanation: "BMI. Body mass index. It tells you if you have a healthy weight compared to your height."

Once I heard the affirmative "Huh" from Chris, I continued. "She wants to take him to ICLI meetings. I'm just trying to help him out. If you notice anything with him, let me know."

"Will do," she affirmed. "I'll see you later. I've got to mop up some noodles."

About five seconds after I hung up the phone it rang again. It was another one of Davis' secretaries.

"Hi, may I speak to Finn," she said.

I told her she had me.

"Hi Finn," she breezed. "This is Jane at the clinic. Dr. Jones asked me to give you a call. He had a couple of big injuries come in a while ago. He's running behind but was wondering if he could call you this evening." She sounded way cooler than his other secretary.

"Thanks Jane," I answered. "Could you tell him not to worry about it? I'll get in touch over the weekend. It's not urgent."

"Sure thing Finn," she said, signing off. "I'll let him know."

"Thanks again," I finished. "I appreciate you calling."

"My pleasure," she popped back.

And that's how to talk to a teenager.

CHAPTER 13

Right after supper, Charlie and Chris came over for our usual Friday night movie night. It's kind of a family night, but we're usually allowed to invite a friend or two.

Fiona had her best friend Vicky over. They do dance and go to school together, so they might as well be joined at the hip.

The drag with Vicky is that she does not seem to take her eyes off me. Trust me, it's the pits, not to mention a little creepy, to have your sister's friend always staring at you. I feel like I'm being followed by the paparazzi or something. I asked Fi why she does it, and she just giggled. Anyway, I guess now I know what it's like to be a celebrity. In a bad way.

Tonight we were watching an old classic: Star Wars. We were all cozy (translation: squashed) in our den, and we had the usual popcorn and soda (which we call pop in Canada), plus a warm batch of brownies.

Usually Mom is the organic and natural food

queen. But she loosens up for movie night. (Saying that, who knows what was in the brownies. Something healthy, I'm sure. And the soda was some kind of all-natural concoction. We sometimes have a 'don't ask, don't tell' policy.)

I hate to say it, but I had one eye on the t.v. and one eye on Charlie. I guess I had never noticed how many times he dips into the snacks. The other thing is, he found his spot on the couch and did not move.

At all.

Everyone else got up at least once to stretch or get some water or something, but Charlie just positioned himself by the snack table and got into semi-hibernation mode.

Chris was a different story. She is always fidgeting and tonight was no different. Interesting.

And Fiona... Holy smokes. Mom asked her for the fifth time if she'd like a brownie, and for the fifth time she said no thanks, as if Mom had offered her a rock to eat. Then she actually got down on the floor at one point and started stretching and doing these V-sits.

"Workin' on your abs, Fi?" I asked. (I had decided to go easy on the Fifi thing. Mom and Dad seemed worried about her eating, and I was beginning to wonder if she was sick.)

Mom looked over at her, then gave her 'get a load of this' look and head tilt to Dad. (Not in a good way.)

I glanced over at Charlie a few times, to see if he had even changed position. Each time I did, the only movement was Vicky, putting her hands over her face to cover the fact she was staring at me. Ugh.

At one point I looked over and Charlie had actually sunken into recliner mode. Without the recliner.

Chris, who was up to grab a tissue, tapped me and motioned with a quick head flick. I had to admit, Charlie was so sluggish looking, he was reminding me a little too much of Jabba the Hutt.

I kept going back to Dad's comment about balance. I was seeing a relationship here.

Man, I felt like Charlie was my little science experiment. I would continue gathering info tomorrow. For now, it was time to focus on Luke, Hans Solo, Princess Leia and a big furry dude named Chewbacca.

CHAPTER 14

The next morning, I woke up, stretched, and patted Ralph, who was loyally snoozing at around knee level on my bed. I heard voices downstairs. (We have an old-fashioned heating system, so the ducts are awesome for listening in on top-secret conversations.)

Ralph inched up toward my pillow for a snuggle. I scratched behind his ears and he gave me his 'I love you man' look.

"Come on Ralphie," I coaxed.

I got up and padded downstairs, with Ralph right beside me, his pawnails clicking on the wood.

As expected, I found Mom, Dad, and Davis sitting at the kitchen table with coffee and a basket of muffins. I could see and hear them before they saw me.

"It's absolutely ridiculous," Dad was saying. "Why don't you let me talk to her?"

"Let's both talk to her. After I have a little word with her dance teacher." Mom said the last part in a pretty menacing way. (The only thing worse than having a 'chit chat' with Mom is having a 'word' with her.)

"I think that's a smart idea. Just don't get all grizzly-mama on her now, Katie," joked Davis. "Or at least invite me if you do."

I emerged from the hallway.

"Hey big guy," Dad boomed, as I walked in with Ralph. I waved weakly, my eyes still bleary.

Of course Ralph bolted right over to Davis who, for a big guy, can talk in a surprisingly coochy-coo voice to my dog. Ralph loves him.

"What's the Ralphie sayin'? What's my sweet buddy sayin'," Davis started in as Ralph slobbered all over him. Davis is a tall, built, stylin' African American man and he's one of the most well-read and eloquent people I know. However, when he gets around Ralph, he basically turns to mush. It always cracks me up.

"Good morning sleepyhead," Mom purred brightly. I looked at the kitchen clock.

"It's eight thirty," I countered. Not exactly sleeping til noontime.

Davis grinned broadly. "Hey Finn, how are you?"

I ran my hand through my bedhead. "Hey Davis. Great. How are you?"

He stuck out his fist and we bumped.

I've got to tell you, Davis is at the top of my 'coolest people I know' list. He's always Mr. Laid Back, he's a good athlete and was a super fast sprinter. Plus, he's a volunteer coach with our track club. Just a good karma kind of dude. He grew up in a pretty tough area in Baltimore, but he kept his nose clean (his words, not mine) and worked hard. (Plus he helped me on an African American studies project a while back, so he just moved up on my cool list.)

"I'm great man. Thanks," he said, still smiling. Davis is always pretty upbeat. "So, I got your message yesterday, and your dad and I were talking earlier about your interest in weight and BMI."

I got some orange juice and grabbed a seat at the table with them.

"Yeah, my friend Charlie," I started.

Davis nodded. "Well, you know, I can't talk to you about specific patients because that's sort of confidential. Privacy and all."

"Cool. I understand," I nodded. Oh yeah, I forgot about that whole doctor-patient confidentiality thing.

"But," he held up his index finger and tapped it on his nose, "I can give you some general information. You know... what I would suggest for a young man who wants to get to a healthy weight." He raised one eyebrow. "Instead of going to weight control meetings with older people."

Aha, so Dad had filled him in. I took a slug of my juice and grabbed a muffin as Davis continued.

"Now, for a young, otherwise healthy guy, a big thing is education. He's got to learn about portion control, being active, etc. The other big deal is parental involvement. The parents have to be on board to support him in his choices. Because the bottom line is, the guy wouldn't need a diet. Diets are often temporary. He would need a lifestyle change," Davis concluded.

It was my turn to raise my eyebrows. "So, there are alternatives to ICLI," I asked without actually asking.

Davis nodded. "It's all about,"

"Balance," I finished.

He fist-bumped me.

"Basically ICLI is education and support. They teach things like healthy eating, ways to control how much you're eating, and active lifestyle," Davis went on. "If a young guy had other resources, he could see a nutritionist. He could even see a personal trainer for the activity portion, if he had the monetary back-up."

(This cracked me up. Of course, we all knew who we were talking about, and Davis knows that Charlie's family is loaded. However, we all continued the charade.)

"A family doctor, such as myself, could set all that up, if the young man's parent brought him into the office," he cleared his throat. "Again."

Davis leaned back. "A guy should feel comfortable talking to his doctor about this stuff," he added. "It's all cool."

I grabbed another muffin. Sometimes Mom's muffins were like horse feed (all oats and fiber), but these were really delicious.

"Okay," I played along, speaking in a top-secret tone. "So if, say, the random young gentleman came back in with his parent, and they were aware of and open to alternatives, you would be able to discuss those options to set up the afore-mentioned-"

I stopped and looked directly at Davis.

"What were we just talking about?"

Davis sat up laughing. "No problem. Yeah, we could do something for the random young gentleman." He looked at Mom and Dad. "I know some excellent trainers and nutritionists," he said, looking from one to the other. "You both must have some suggestions too."

They both nodded to Davis and me.

"There's a German PhD student at UNC's exercise physiology department who specializes in personal training for younger folks, who I've heard amazing things about," Dad said.

For some reason, I got a mental picture of some hulking bodybuilder named Hans. Or Franz. My second mental picture was Charlie laying under a huge barbell. Not good.

"Hmm," I thought out loud. "I don't know if Charlie wants some hulk of a trainer.

"Well Finn," Davis piped up, "There are lots of choices. There are a ton of amazing personal trainers who can help Ch- er I mean a brother, out."

"That's fantastic Davis," I said, pumped up. "Thanks a lot."

"No sweat, Finn," Davis replied, high fiving me. "Hey, how's the tennis?"

"Awesome," I said. My usual answer.

"Right on," Davis replied, winking. "Don't get too good man. I won't be able to play you."

I laughed but I had to make tracks. I had to tell

Charlie the good news. Then it was just a matter of talking to his mom. We were in business. But first, my favorite part of the weekend: tennis.

Mom looked at me. "I've got to pop by the studio," she informed me. "How are you getting to tennis?"

I pointed at my feet. "With Lefty and Righty here," I returned. "Why, you want to drive me?" I gave her my most endearing smile.

"Sure," she smiled back. "If you don't mind dropping by Fiona's dance class first with me."

"I'll walk thanks."

Davis got up to grab more coffee. Like everyone, he feels really at home at our place, which is cool.

He patted my shoulder on the way by and I nearly spit out my juice. Obviously Davis is still doing some upper body strength training. "You running the 400 for spring track? Everyone knows sprinters get all the chicks."

Dad fake-coughed and they laughed.

"Okay boys," Mom piped in. I looked at her, thinking she was talking to Ralph and me. Oh, she was talking to them.

Ralph looked up at me with his suck-up eyes. I looked at my watch. Tennis was at nine thirty. "Uh oh, I've got to get Ralph out," I remembered.

Dad laughed. "We took him to the park. He ran off-leash with us on the trails."

"But he was sleeping in his usual spot on my bed when I woke up," I protested.

They laughed and Mom shrugged. "Smart dog."

Right. Ralphie had had his morning romp. Things were looking good for Charlie. We were in business, after I hit the courts. I mean, even investigators have got to have some fun.

CHAPTER 15

Tennis was awesome as usual.

Mom and Dad first put me in lessons way back when I was five, but we used to bat the ball around with the racket when I could barely walk.

They don't push any sports with us, except this. Mom says she wants to be able to play at least one sport with us. (You don't want to see her on the basketball court. Very messy.) And they want us to learn some lifetime sports, so supposedly we can play when we're ninety.

Saturday morning tennis is particularly cool because Tom and Xavier are in it. After we play and get cleaned up, we usually head downtown and grab a bite to eat at this little diner. Chris is also here but they separate guys from girls. Lame if you ask me. Chris can whip most guys' butts at tennis.

Today we were working on smash. The smash looks like a serve. You smash the ball (the ball is actually fine) when it gets lobbed over to you. When you smash it, the ball goes careening back to your opponent's court at a crazy angle, and they usually can't get it. That's the theory anyway.

Halfway though the lesson, Rob, our instructor, brought out 'the Lobster'. No, it's not a tasty crustacean from Nova Scotia. It's this automatic tennis ball shooter. (The name is a play on the whole 'lob' aspect of tennis, since the machine lobs balls at whatever angle and speed you want.)

Every time Rob gets out the Lobster, we get the lecture on paying attention and not goofing off.

The old 'we don't want someone to lose an eye' speech.

Rob's a good guy, just a little serious sometimes. But I guess you have to be when you have eight guys and a lot of potential projectiles.

So here we were in our little half circle, while Rob stood in front of us, giving us the 'if you get hurt fooling around, I'm gonna kill you' talk.

Rob rolled the Lobster to the middle of one side of the court, adjusted the speed, and aimed it at us. He came over and smashed a couple of balls to demonstrate. He's an awesome player, so his technique is perfect, and he's Mr. Calm on the court.

Then he stood well off to the side. The balls started popping out and lobbing into the air, and we had to take turns at the front of the line, smashing them back over the net.

The first round went great. Most of us got up to the line, focused, and connected with the ball.

Rob stood there nodding. "Nice, nice," he said. Then when one of us hit a particularly good one, he got all pumped and started yelling stuff like,

"Yeah! Dominate!"

After a few rounds we were starting to loosen up with it and get cocky. The balls were coming pretty fast, and to two different spots on the court. We were stepping up and doing our best "Hiyugh!" as we smashed it, trying to be all menacing, like some of the pros.

We finished the lesson with a game of 'poison ball', where you have to run back and forth across the court and try not to get hit with a ball. Rob aims the Lobster down, on crazy mode, and the balls shoot out at random speeds and locations. This is when he really loosens up and gets fun. He always plays it with us and it's hilarious to see him leaping around as he runs, trying to avoid the balls.

We had a great game and we were tired after. That good kind of tired. I looked over. Tom was whispering something to Xavier, and Xav was laughing, twitching around, still looking like the Energizer Bunny. Man, that guy never stops.

CHAPTER 16

We walked over to Anna's Diner after the lesson. It's about a ten-minute walk from the tennis center. Tom, Xavier and I always get a booth, and Chris sits with a few of the girls in her tennis class. Sometimes we get tables beside each other and we all hang out. The girls who do tennis are pretty cool.

Anna's Diner is actually an old classic train diner, with an extra part built on. We always sit in the old part, and usually Anna herself is there.

Anna would make a great tennis player: She's tough as nails, and has forearms that are huge, and she keeps on swinging… a spatula that is. I think she went to the School of Hard Knocks, grew up on the wrong side of the tracks, and every other hard-luck analogy you could make. But she always has a smile on her face. So, besides having the best breakfast in town, everyone likes to go to Anna's because you sort of want to support someone who kicks butt.

Today we had back-to-back booths. We ordered our usual: fruit pancakes. Anna makes them with all these whole grains and other healthy stuff. They're hearty and really delicious. Today's choice was blueberry – a classic.

Anna came out of the kitchen with the usual grin. "Are you going to get me tickets when you all make it to Wimbledon?"

"Hey Anna. Heck yeah, if you make us pancakes for our pre-game meal," Tom joked back.

"Yeah seriously," Xav added. And he *was* serious.

We were still all pumped up from tennis, but Xavier was squirming around like a ferret on pure sugar. Not that this was anything new. I was just noticing more.

The pancakes were out quick, along with tall, frosty glasses of milk. Once the plates hit the table and we picked up our forks, all conversation stopped. Sometimes you don't realize how hungry you are.

"You going to Charlie's tonight?" Tom asked, after a couple of minutes.

I nodded, my mouth full of juicy warm pancakes.

"It'll be fun," Tom followed up. We were going to sleep out in the pool house, and have access to the indoor pool also.

I looked up as I reached for a little syrup. Xavier was already halfway through his stack. Man, that guy can eat. For a wiry guy, you really do wonder about the hollow leg concept. Seriously, where does he put it?

Once we were most of the way through the

pancakes, conversation resumed. It was the usual: sports, what everyone was up to this weekend, more sports, the project we had due for school, and yes, more sports.

"You should get Charlie out for tennis," Xavier said. They know he's my best friend, but they pal around with him too.

"Yeah," Tom replied. "I don't know why he hasn't ever signed up. The guy's got his own tennis court."

"I think he's had a few private lessons," I answered.

"Yeah, he has one this morning," Tom said.

"Really?"

"Yeah," Tom continued. "He told me yesterday. He made a point of telling me that he had this big tennis session this morning. Maybe we've been razzing him too much about coming out with us. He seemed kind of defensive." He paused.

Xavier nodded. "He made a point of telling me he was going to be playing all morning too. He's probably still on the court."

"Hmm," I said, half to myself.

Tom, the social butterfly shook his head. "Yeah but that's not the same as hitting with your friends."

"Yeah," I said, nodding. I've asked Charlie about doing tennis with us but he never sounds too keen. I looked at my watch. "I've got to get home and call Charlie now."

Tom was draining his milk and Xavier was vacuuming up the last of his pancakes.

I turned around and flicked the back of Chris's

head. Yeah, I know: subtle. "You walking?"

Chris gave me her trademark miffed look: lips puckered to the side and eyebrows pushed together. "Ex-squeeze me?"

"Ready?" I said, holding out my hands, giving her my 'what?' look as the other girls humphed. Sensitive much?

"Okay, one minute," she said. She turned around and I turned back to the guys, nice and casual. I know how to talk to chicks. Just treat 'em like guys.

"So," I started.

Agh! I felt an icy cold napkin ball, beaned at the back of my head. Special.

I turned around. Chris cocked her head at me sweetly and said, "Ready."

Okay, point taken. I put some money down for a tip and got up. "See you guys," I signed off.

Tom leaned back. "Dad's picking us up in about five minutes if you guys want a lift."

"Nah, I'm good thanks," I said. "I'm so full, the pancakes feel like they're expanding in my stomach. I've got to burn these off."

Lightbulb.

Now I get that saying. Yeah! I had to burn off the calories, the fuel. By getting up and moving, I was going to burn more calories, and faster... and feel better. That's what Dad was talking about! And it's not that hard. In fact, now that I think of it, it's easier than Charlie thinks.

We signed off with our buddies, paid at the cash register, waved thanks to Anna and walked out.

CHAPTER 17

As we meandered toward home (meandering was the best I could do on a full stomach), we talked a bit about tennis.

And then we didn't talk. Chris is pretty cool that way. If she doesn't have anything to say, she doesn't try to do fill-in conversation. She's okay with a little silence.

I was distracted, thinking about Fiona and Charlie.

Out of the blue, I asked, "Does Fiona look skinnier to you?"

Chris looked surprised at the question. She thought about it for a minute.

"Actually Finn, yeah, she does look like she's lost some weight," she replied. "What's up? Is she okay?"

"I think my folks are worried that she's trying to lose weight for dance," I confided. "That's kind of a secret."

Chris shook her head and gave me a wry smile. "But she's tiny. It's good they're on it," she said.

"Want me to talk to her?"

(Fiona kind of looks up to Chris, and Chris treats her like the little sister she doesn't have. I have offered to donate her. Just kidding!)

"Hmm. No. Not yet anyway," I said softly. "Thanks though."

She took a breath like she was going to say something, then she stopped. She was thinking about something.

We walked along. Finally, I said, "What?" (I know, not the most warm and fuzzy approach.)

She looked at me. "What what?"

I had to laugh. "You were just going to say something. You're not going to start keeping secrets from your favorite pal now are you?" I grinned.

Chris hesitated.

"Just tell me," I urged.

"Well, I didn't really tell you this last year, but remember when I had the crazy assistant soccer coach?"

"Yeah."

"Yeah, well he took me aside and said that if I wanted to play really high caliber soccer, I should lose a few pounds."

"What?!"

Yes, I was incredulous. Chris is the fittest, most solid girl I know. (She's also the prettiest, and I say that objectively.) She's the best player, by far, on her team.

Chris nodded. "Yep," she affirmed. "At first I felt pretty bad. Then I talked to Mom and she was really upset. She called our head coach. It turns out he was talking to a few girls about their weight. Girls who were healthy. Don't say anything but I think that's why the assistant got fired."

I looked at Chris. "Why didn't you tell me?"

She was a little sheepish. "I guess I was embarrassed."

I didn't quite know what to say. "Yeah well, I think you look great. And you're good." (Did that even make sense?) Then, for good measure, I gave her a soft punch on the shoulder.

She glanced at me and smiled. "Thanks Finn," she said sweetly, punching me back. (Ouch, my shoulder.)

Suddenly she grinned. "Geez that Xavier can eat," she laughed. I nodded. We picked up the pace a little. "Hey," she added, "Did you notice Charlie chowing down last night?"

I nodded my head. "I know." I paused. "You know, he and Xav are the only ones who can finish Anna's pancakes."

We walked for a minute. Out of the blue, I had a brilliant (as Charlie would say) idea.

"Hey Chris," I started, pumped. "Want to come with me and do some reconnaissance?"

"Some what?!"

I gave her my 'you've got to be kidding, you think you're an A student?' look. Then I realized, I only know the word from reading so many spy books.

"Come and help me investigate something," I prodded. "I want to check out Charlie's tennis lesson."

"What? Why?" It was her incredulous/'this is

a bad idea' tone.

"Come on woman. Any good investigator knows that he has to observe his subject. I want to see how much he's exercising, but without him thinking I'm spying on him."

"Which you totally are."

"Not the point."

Off her look, I said, "We'll be quick, I promise."

So we took a couple of shortcuts and came onto the grounds near Charlie's tennis court.

"Get down," I whispered to Chris, as I dropped and slithered around a bush on my stomach. Luckily my tennis racket was over my back.

"Are you for real," she started to say as I reached up for her arm and tugged.

Not a good idea. She fell, landing on me.

"Ouch," she growled.

"Sorry, sorry," I said. "But you're not exactly a bag of marshmallows."

Hmm, that didn't come out right. She gave me the lasers with her eyes. Oops.

"Sorry Chris," I followed up. "You okay?"

She nodded then focused on what I was looking at:

Charlie's instructor was showing him serves. Charlie sat on the bench at the side of the court.

Chris and I looked at each other. I put my hand up, pointed at her, then me, pointed forward, then tugged on my ear, put my finger to my lips, and did a swirly motion with my hand.

She gave me her one eyebrow raise look.

Okay, I admit, I didn't know what the last

swirly signal was for. I just got carried away. This was kind of fun.

We slithered forward to the next bush. Now we could hear them.

"Charlie, you sure you don't want to at least try a few more serves?" It was his tennis instructor. "That won't hurt your knee."

"I think I should get some ice on this knee, and I'm really knackered," Charlie replied.

Chris nudged me. "He's always making excuses to get out of things early," she whispered.

I nodded. Then I put two fingers in front of my eyes and pointed them at Charlie. Chris rolled her eyes.

"Let's pick up these balls then," the instructor said, trying to keep a positive tone.

They both went around with a basket each and popped the balls in. Charlie was moving like a snail, and not a happy snail.

I looked at Chris again as they walked off the court, toward the house. I was about to give another signal when I felt the water.

The sprinklers! I forgot they were on timers!

We got up and were about to start running, when Chris half screamed "Ahhh!"

Yes, the water was cold, but quite refreshing. The tennis instructor and Charlie were starting to turn around.

I had to act on lightning fast reflexes. I pushed her into another shrub.

"Ow!"

"Sorry sorry," I whispered. "I didn't want them to see us."

I lifted my head to the top of the shrub. They had turned back around again and were going to the house.

"Yeah, well maybe they want to see this!" Chris lunged and jumped on me. She moved, remarkably, like a jungle cat. I was impressed until she slammed into me. It was kind of playful, and yet kind of hurt. Mental note: Don't mess with Chris.

CHAPTER 18

We were walking back toward Chris' house. I was a little sore from her ambush.

"So, obviously Charlie isn't exercising when he says he does," I stated. "Or at least he's overestimating how much exercise he's getting."

Chris nodded. "And he's eating way too much," she agreed. "I mean, Xavier eats a lot too, but he's always moving. He needs the extra energy," she added.

"I got curious about Charlie's situation," Chris said. "So I looked it-"

"And Charlie doesn't," I stated, snapping my fingers. I stopped in my tracks and looked at Chris.

"Doesn't what? Chris said.

"Doesn't move as much," I said, my eyes lighting up. I clapped my hands, the lightbulb lit again. "It's the balance thing again! He doesn't need the extra energy. And doesn't need the extra food!"

This was all coming together!

"Okay man, don't lay an egg on me," Chris bounced back.

In the middle of my Thomas Edison moment, I looked at Chris. "Lay an egg?"

Chris looked at me and shrugged. Sometimes, I swear, we bicker like an old married couple.

"What I had started to say, before you interrupted me," Chris scolded me, "Is that I looked up BMI after we got off the phone yesterday."

I nodded, humoring her. I had already done this legwork.

"And I messed up initially," she continued. "I started to Google it, but I forgot the last letter." Chris gave me a playful slap with the back of her hand, laughing. "Do you know what BM means?" Without waiting for my reply: "Bowel movement! Isn't that gross? It means have a crap!"

I half-laughed, half-cringed. Like I say, a girly-girl Chris was not. "Well Sherlock, that's a really extraordinary piece of detective work. Thanks very much. Now I have a code abbreviation when I want to poop."

Still laughing, Chris re-focused. "Right. The point. I ended up looking up BMR, instead of BMI. The remarkable thing is that they're related."

We were nearing Chris' house. "It's still on my computer. I'll show you," she said. "Do you have a few minutes?"

I looked at my watch. I had to get home, take Ralph out, call Charlie, and I was going to get some info that Callie had promised me, but I still had a few minutes. I nodded. "Yeah okay, thanks."

Chris led the way up her walkway and into her house. She yelled out, "Anyone home?"

"Hey Chrissie!" It was her brother Sam, calling from upstairs. "Just studying in my room!"

"I'm just going to show Finn something," Chris bellowed back.

"Hey Sam," I shouted upward.

"Hey Finn," Sam yelled back.

Luckily, I get along really well with Chris's big brothers. I wouldn't want to be the guy picking her up for a date. They are protective with a capital P.

Chris's computer was set up at a little workstation in the kitchen. I could smell the tomato sauce from the noodles that must have been all over her kitchen yesterday.

"You want anything?" she asked. The thought of Chris fixing a snack was a little scary, and besides, the pancakes felt like they were still expanding in my stomach. And I wasn't thirsty. I shook my head, said "no thanks" and we sat down.

Chris turned, woke up her computer, and scrolled down the 'history' tab. After she pointed at the 'BM' and snickered, we got down to work.

So here's what we saw:

BMR = basal metabolic rate - The minimum energy the body requires to maintain necessary bodily functions.

Sounds kind of boring, but when we read further, it basically compared the body to a car engine.

Your basal metabolic rate is the calories you burn to keep your body in park; just like a car.

Like, if you were going to lay on the couch and do nothing all day. I never thought about it, but you need energy to keep your heart beating, make new cells, breathe, and all that stuff that you never think about. It hadn't sunken in before, but this was what Cassie had meant when she talked about metabolism.

I looked at Chris. "This is kind of cool, but,"

She interrupted me by pointing to the screen. "This caught my eye for a couple of reasons. I heard one of the teachers complaining to Ms. Mac that her metabolism had slowed down and she was gaining weight."

"Who?"

"Mrs. Adams."

"I think she's the one who's slow. She's like a snail."

Chris wagged her index finger at me. "Precisely!"

She pressed her finger to her pursed lips. It kind of made her look like a (mad) scientist.

I stifled a laugh, mainly because she had a good point. (But she did have a hilarious expression on her face, trying to be so serious and focused. Especially after the 'bowel movement' bit.)

She moved the mouse. "Look at Charlie. He's pretty inactive. His metabolism is probably running at a snail's pace, so he's not burning many calories."

Chris directed me to the screen again. It showed a scale with the heading 'Energy Balance':

Energy Intake
Energy Expenditure (used)
Food you eat BMR, digestion, activity

I looked at the digestion thing. "You burn calories by just eating?"

"Yeah. Well, by digesting what you eat. Although I guess chewing and swallowing would burn a couple of calories. Neat huh? Digestion's a pretty major process," Chris said, turning to me. "Haven't you ever heard that you'll never gain weight by eating celery? Because you actually use more calories to chew and digest it than are in it?"

I gave my interested shrug/nod/"huh" combination.

"So, see here." Chris pointed to the screen, to the picture of a scale tipped towards food. "Charlie doesn't have a good energy balance. He's eating more energy, in food, than he's burning off. So he's gaining weight."

"So he's eating way too many calories. And he's running his engine on low, hardly burning any calories, and all that extra energy is getting stored as fat," I finished. "It's all coming back to having balance."

Chris sat back. "Precisely."

(Yes, I know Dad had told me this before, but, and I hate to say this, I wasn't really listening. Or should I say, believing.)

I nodded my head at her. "See doll, this is why I keep you around," I said in my best movie tough guy voice, "You've got smarts."

Chris raised her eyebrows. "Stop watching

mob movies, boy."

She got up. "If he watches what he eats, and just seriously moves more, he'll start losing weight. He doesn't have to start a new sport or go to a camp. He simply has to burn more calories than he eats, every day."

She sat on the counter. "He has to tip the scale the other way. Then, once he's at a good weight, he has to keep it even."

I got up. "This is very straightforward," I stated. "No wonder Davis was talking about lifestyle change."

It was all coming together.

I heard a 'ting' from my pocket. I took out my phone and looked. It was another novel length text from Mom.

Hi Finn,
I'm just wondering where you are. Did you go to Anna's? Charlie called, looking for you. I hope you had fun at tennis. Ralph says Hi. Love, Mom ☺

Mental note: Must teach Mom the difference between texting and writing an English essay.

At Chris's. C U soon. ☺Finn

And another 'ting'. This one from Charlie.

Where R U?

I texted back.

With Chris. Going 2 C Cassie.

'Ting'.

Meet U there!

Oh yeah, you know about Charlie's little - okay huge - crush on Cassie. For a guy who does drama, he doesn't do a great job of hiding it either. Every time Cassie comes over, Charlie mysteriously shows up, and every opportunity he has to see her, he's on it. He was just voted 'Most Devoted Fan' of the high school girls' volleyball team.

I got up and stretched. "Okay thanks Chris," I started to say, while yawning at the same time. Chris caught me in mid-yawn with an abs grab. So it came out more like "Okay thanks Cree-ahhh!"

Chris started laughing, with a very insincere "Sorry, couldn't resist," between cackles.

Then, as I grabbed my racket and headed for the door, she stopped, sniffed, and asked, "Can you still smell lasagna?"

CHAPTER 19

Cassie's house was only a couple of minute walk from Chris's, and my pancakes were digesting, so I picked it up from a meander to a stroll.

I had texted Cassie about that info she had. Even though things were coming together, I believe in being thorough.

As I turned the corner, I saw Charlie leaning, nonchalantly against a tree, trying to be Mr. Cool.

I walked up and said "Hey".

Charlie "Hey"d me back.

I wanted to see if he'd mention the tennis lesson. "What'd you do this morning?"

Charlie stretched his arms out. "Big tennis session this morning. I'm zonked."

When I didn't answer, he followed up. "Just exhausted."

Uh huh.

We walked up to Cassie's front porch. I had to take a deep breath to brace myself from laughing, because I knew what was coming.

I knocked and Cassie opened the door. "Hey

Finn! Hey Charlie, what a surprise." (It totally wasn't.)

I gave her my knowing smile. She winked at me.

Charlie had his eyes half closed and his chin up, and was kind of biting his bottom lip… I think in an attempt to look cool…?!

"Heh Casseh," he said, trying so hard to be casual that he kind of got the first word sounds out but nothing else. (It sound like "hh Cah-ssehh".)

Cassie smiled. "Come on in guys. Can I get you anything?"

Charlie started to say something but food meant a longer visit, and I had to get home to Ralph.

"No thanks Cass," I trumpeted. "We're good."

Charlie looked at me, miffed. "I've got to get home and get Ralphie out," I explained.

Cassie went to the kitchen island and picked up a plate of cookies. "You sure? I just baked these."

Charlie looked at her like she was a goddess. "Well, maybe just one," he replied, still in his forced casual, I'm-not-going-to-annunciate-clearly mode. He grabbed two cookies together as if they were one, and took a little nibble. "Wow, these are amazing Cass-sehh."

Cassie looked at me. "You sure Finn? They're pretty healthy, and they're even warm."

"Trust me, I'd love one, but I'm still too full," I explained. "Anna's pancakes."

"Oh. Say no more. The volleyball team goes there sometimes after practice," she commiserated. "Want me to wrap a couple up for you for later?" She put the plate back down.

"Yeah sure. Thanks Cass," I replied.

Cassie went to a drawer. "Sit down guys." She got out some plastic wrap. "You know Finn, that's good you didn't take a cookie if you didn't want one now. In the project I did on," she glanced at Charlie, "what we talked about, I learned how a lot of us eat due to peer pressure and other reasons. Like me just pushing my cookies on you guys. Sorry."

Charlie had somehow finished the cookie sandwich and was gazing adoringly at Cassie.

"No way, are you kidding? Thanks," I said to Cassie as she handed me the little sweet package.

"Okay Charlie," I continued loudly, snapping him out of it. "I really have to get back."

Charlie jumped a little then got up. Cassie handed me a folder. "There's some neat stuff in there. Interesting information. Good luck."

Cassie walked us to the door. "So Charlie, how's your acting going?"

I could just about hear his heart racing. "It's fantastic. We're going to do a musical in the spring," Charlie answered, more coherent this time. "Guys and Dolls!"

Acting is Charlie's thing for sure. You can tell because he kind of forgets himself when he talks about it.

"Wow," she said, genuinely impressed. Then to me, "Let me know when you get tickets and we'll go see it with your family."

I nodded. She just made his month.

Cassie opened the door. "Thanks again Cas," I said, holding up the folder. "See you around."

"See you guys," Cassie said smiling, and she winked at us. I sensed a shudder go through Charlie, and then he found his words again. "See yeh Cas-sehh."

Hmm, must work on Charlie's casual approach.

CHAPTER 20

As Charlie and I walked back toward my place, I filled him in on what I had learned.

"It's like you talked about with being on stage. Balance is the key thing here."

I looked at him to let that sink in. No response.

"You just need to balance out how many calories you're taking in with what you're burning," I told him earnestly. "But for the next while, you have to create a negative balance. You have to burn more calories than you eat. So you're going to have to do some exercise."

"I exercise."

(My little reconnaissance mission with Chris had told me otherwise. Charlie was just showing up, and calling it exercise.)

"Well, Charlie, you want to do something where you'll really move," I told him, trying to put it delicately.

Charlie groaned and shook his head. "I don't know mate. I think this is all genetic."

I rolled my eyes toward him. "Trust me Charlie, it's not genetic." (If you met Beatrice you'd know why, and Mr. Bienenstock looks like a pro football player.)

I paused, so he could take it all in. "You've got to see Davis again. He can set you up with a nutritionist and a trainer if that'll help. Dad knows some German dude."

Charlie looked at me in horror. "Are you kidding me? I can't have some big German ex-weightlifter telling me to do more crunches!" He slowed down. "I'm doomed," he groaned dramatically.

Charlie seemed to slow down while we were even talking about exercise.

"The other thing is, everything hurts when I exercise. My knees, my feet," he trailed off.

"Yeah but they'll probably feel better if you take a little load off them and strengthen up your legs," I advised. "I mean, you just have to get more active to start. No one's asking you to do a triathlon."

Charlie was looking down as we walked, really bummed out.

"Your first step," I told him firmly, "is to talk to Beatrice.

Charlie groaned again.

"I can't talk to Beatrice," he exclaimed. "She has her mind made up. You know what she's like!"

"Charlie, you asked me to help you out, and I'm trying," I said, putting my hand on his shoulder. "But there's no magic remedy to losing the weight. There's no pill or tonic. It's got to be you."

He looked at the ground. "Maybe ICLI wouldn't be so bad," he muttered.

CHAPTER 21

Charlie and I parted ways at the path behind my house. I had asked him if he wanted to take Ralph to the park with me, but he claimed he was too tired.

See, that would have been an opportunity. Be active. Burn a few more calories. Rev up the motor.

After I threw Ralph's ball approximately a million times, we came home and had a snack. My new favorite is peanut butter and banana rolled up in a tortilla. Whoever invented the peanut butter and banana combo is a genius.

I sat down at the kitchen table and started to chow down while Ralph lay down beside me to mooch. I flipped through the mail: a couple of bills, a dance magazine, and *LL Bean* and *Land's End* catalogues.

Hmm, the new *Men's Health* had arrived. I flipped through it. I could hear Mom and Dad in the next room, talking in their 'serious' voices.

I didn't want to interrupt but I totally wanted

to be nosy. I got a glass and held the open end against the wall. I stuck my ear against the other end and listened. (I saw somebody do this on an old spy movie.) Not exactly Dolby digital sound but pretty good! Seriously, try it sometime. You can totally eavesdrop on somebody talking in another room!

"Her teacher didn't seem to think there was a problem," Mom was saying. "She says she has huge potential and has a ballerina's body."

"Yeah, well she hasn't seen her refusing to eat these days," Dad concurred. "Doesn't she get that you have to be strong to dance? That they need that fuel?"

"Obviously not."

"Did she say anything else?"

"She told me she had a class starting and that she didn't really have time to talk about the choices Fiona makes at home," Mom said, clearly miffed.

And a well-placed "hmm" from Dad. Maybe I'd get back to my snack. I started to take my ear away-

Mom went on.

"So then I said, 'Well, clearly you do have time to talk about the choices the girls make at home, because you seem to be telling them to avoid things like milk, cheese, bread, and fruit. And that's getting into some bad territory here.'"

I put the glass back against the wall. Mom was getting into her backcountry drawl. She was fired up.

"Great approach," Dad agreed.

But Mom didn't stop there. "I said, 'I have my Masters in this area and frankly, asking girls to starve themselves to be as thin as possible is a very dangerous path to start them on. If I remember my basics, dancers also need to be strong.' Then do you know what she said to me?"

Ooh, Mom was getting into cobra mode.

"She said, 'If Fiona chooses to eat like a cow, she can go right ahead, but she'll never make it as a ballet dancer.' Can you freaking believe that?!"

And a pause. Dad treads lightly when Mom gets into backcountry cobra mode and starts using words like 'freaking' and 'frig'.

"That's when I said, "Well guess what? I'm making a choice right now. I'm taking Fiona home and she is never coming back! And you can take your advice and stick it-"

"Okay! Yeah…" Darn, Dad was trying to calm her down just when this was getting good. (Mom is so chilled out all the time, I find it hilarious when she gets riled up.)

"Well," Dad said, in his calm tone.

"Oh no, it didn't end there," Mom continued. "She had the nerve to say 'You are making a huge mistake. She could have been someone.'"

A little "uh oh" from Dad.

"So I said, 'How dare you. Trust me, she is somebody now! And she's going to be someone long after you've withered away to nothing! You will never tell my daughter what to do.'"

(A pause.)

"Then I stormed out with Fiona dragging her feet behind me," Mom finished.

All I heard was a "wow" from Dad. Then a chuckle. "Davis was right. You are a mama bear," Dad said gently. (He probably didn't want to rile her up more.) "You did the right thing Katie. You know you did."

Then Mom added, "So now Fiona won't talk to me. She is furious. I didn't mean to embarrass her, but that couldn't continue. Plus it felt good though to tell that woman a thing or two."

I took the glass down quickly. They might come walking back to the kitchen at any moment.

Oh man, Fiona was going to be brutal to be around for the next while. Geez, I did feel really bad for her. I mean, dancing is a big deal to her. Huge. Kind of like her whole life. I'd go up and check in on her after.

I put the glass away and sat down at the table.

I opened up the folder Callie had given me, and scanned some of the pages. There was some good info for keeping in a healthy weight zone. Lots of the tips were things we already do.

Callie also had some notes on really simple stuff, like little stuff you can do every day to burn more calories. Exercise physiologists studied people while they were standing, sitting, and laying down. Standing up and moving around is the best, but if you even sit up while you're watching t.v., and get up a couple of times, you use more energy than when you're laying there like a log.

I closed the folder and patted Ralph.

Poor Fiona. Now I understood why Mom and Dad kept asking about snacks and were so concerned with her eating enough. It was all a matter of balance for her too. She had tipped the scale the other way and she needed to even things out.

I got a glass of moo juice (milk) and opened up the folder again.

Callie also had a neat article. Literally! Get this: There's this thing called NEAT that researchers are studying: **N**on-**E**xercise **A**ctivity **T**hermogenesis. This is a ridiculously awesomely complicated term for fidgeting. (I put it in my notebook, if you want to have a look.)

I sat back. It was all coming together! It was even easier than I originally thought it would be.

I had to tell Charlie right away. This was not going to be the torture he envisioned. He just had to start moving a bit more and eating appropriate portions. I reached for my phone.

U home?

About ninety seconds later, he replied.

Yep. Playing Wii.

Hmm, maybe he had thought about what I said. Wii is a fairly active video game. I texted back.

C U in 2.

I slipped on my sneakers, grabbed Ralph and pa-toing! I was off through the back door.

I made it to Charlie's in near record time. After getting Ralphie to lay down under one of the shady trees, I knocked on the kitchen door and

Alice let me in.

"Hey Alice," I started. Then I sniffed. "Oh man, not to sound cliché but what smells so good?"

Alice laughed. "Pizza, nachos, apple cake, muffins… It's the food for tonight's sleepover and tomorrow's breakfast, so I'm glad you approve."

"Score," I nodded. "Where's the chief?"

"Master Charlie is in the playroom, playing that 'you' or-"

"Wii?" I asked, stifling a laugh.

"That's it," Alice nodded.

Josie had walked in. "I can summon Master Charlie for you."

(Beatrice must be in the vicinity. Around the house, especially within hearing distance of Charlie's mother, everyone was a little formal.)

"That's okay. I'll go grab him," I answered.

I exited the kitchen and wound my way into his main floor playroom. Charlie was laying on the couch, doing the running course. He was holding the Wii remote in front of him and shaking it up and down. He turned around when I walked in.

"Hey hermano," he crooned as his Mii character puffed along a trail on his massive television. "Check this out, I'm going to break my course record."

I plunked down in another chair. "You're not even vertical man, how can that be fun?" (This was really bringing home the stuff I had just read.)

Charlie shrugged.

I got up and grabbed a remote. "Come on, let's play power tennis."

"Okay." Charlie was like a little sleepy bird in

the nest or something.

Charlie switched it over, and we activated my Mii character, a dark haired dude with a hat and shades.

I got up, ready to start swinging. Facing the television, I shot over, "Ready?"

Charlie shot back, "Let's go!"

Good, he was waking up.

The first point was a long rally, which Charlie won.

"Good one," I said, turning to him. I kept turning. He was still laying on the couch!

"Come on man!" I said, frustrated.

Charlie looked surprised. "What? You can do all these games from the couch."

"But how fun is that? Don't do stuff just because it's the easiest way," I scolded him.

"Well my knees are sore," Charlie started to bluster. I interrupted. "Did you talk to your mom yet?"

"I haven't seen her, and then she had an appointment, and I was going to talk to her after the sleepover, and I haven't even talked to her much since I saw Doc Jones, and I-" Charlie babbled on.

"You want to get weighed in every week and be put on some crazy diet?" I shot at him.

He looked horrified. He sat up, put his elbows on his knees, and ran his fingers through his hair.

I sat across from him and put a hand on his arm. I had seen Dad do that when players were upset, just to chill them out, and bring them down to earth again.

"Charlie man, you asked me to help you, and

I did. But now the ball's in your court. You have got to start moving more. Then you'll lose some weight and feel better. It's not that hard. And it's pretty fun."

No response.

"Come on man," I said gently. "You're my best friend. I want to be able to do stuff with you."

Then he started to sputter, "I bloody well hate sports. I'm tired all the time, and my feet and knees hurt, and I hate the way I look," he said, looking down.

Charlie looked at me kind of blankly. I was searching for the right thing to say. Then he sighed.

"Do you know how embarrassing it is to be fat? To try to do activities with the rest of you? Look at you all, you're all slim and fit and good at everything."

"Good at everything? Charlie, you know I'm only decent at tennis because I love it, so I play and practice so much. And you obviously haven't played soccer with me lately. I'm a spaz," I joked back quietly.

"No you're not," Charlie returned, looking back at me. "And it's football mate," he added, grinning despite himself.

I smiled and nodded but continued as I paced around him a little. "And it's really the opposite. Being active gives you energy."

I let that sink in for a moment before I continued.

"The fitter you are and the more healthy your body weight, the more energy you'll have. Look how tired you are now all the time," I counseled him, and I emphasized, "You feel like crap when you do sports because you're laying around and you're carrying a lot of extra weight around. All – the – time."

Charlie didn't say anything. My little lecture might have been sinking in.

So I kept on truckin'. "And embarrassing? Nobody's judging you. Being overweight doesn't define you Charlie. It's just a state your body is in right now. You have the power to change it. You take ownership of yourself."

(Wow, that was good.)

He just looked at me, half angry, half bummed out.

"No one's asking you to do extra gym classes with that butthead Alan. But don't get all upset, and then do nothing for yourself. Start getting active and that'll shut people like him up." I took a breath. "And who cares what he thinks anyway."

Charlie backed away and slumped on the couch again.

It sucked to have to be this frank with your best friend.

Charlie kind of looked up at a corner of the ceiling. "Would you like me to walk you out?"

Charlie is unfailingly polite, and this was his way of asking me to leave.

"I brought Ralph over," I added hopefully. "Want to come outside?"

"Nah," he replied dully. "I've got to do some homework."

Yeah right.

Now I felt like a rotten guy. I knew it was embarrassing for him now too. But any thought of a magical cure for losing weight and feeling better just wasn't going to happen. He really did have to do this himself.

I got up. Charlie didn't move. "So I'll see you a little later?" I said, in a conciliatory tone.

"Yes, see you then." Charlie looked straight ahead.

I sighed and walked out feeling, well, not so great.

I wound back to the kitchen and saw Alice and Josie folding napkins at one of the huge wooden tables.

I waved.

"See you Finn," they both chimed as I opened the door to go out. They looked at each other. Usually I'm not exactly shy, so they probably wondered if something was wrong. Besides, I had had Ralph leashed to the shady tree for long enough.

When I stepped out, Ralph was happy as a clam, getting his belly rubbed.

"Oh you're such a sweet baby," in that unmistakably royalty-like British accent. "Yes, you adore getting your tummy rubbed."

I cleared my throat, about to say something, but I was kind of speechless.

And then she turned around, stood up, and looked at me. I was face to face with her.

Beatrice.

All five feet of her.

Yes, Beatrice struck fear in our hearts. Yet she's the size of an elf.

"Hello Finn," she said, a little more formally

than a moment ago when she was fawning over Ralph. "I presumed you were around here somewhere. How are you?"

I straightened up automatically. (Habit.)

"Hi Mrs. Bienenstock, I'm fine thanks" I stuttered. Then, annunciating more clearly, "I'm sorry for bringing Ralph over."

She laughed. "Whatever for?"

She thought for a moment. "Oh yes, well it's only Mr. Bienenstock that's allergic. And Josie. I love dogs. I grew up with Labradors."

"Wow, really?" I was impressed.

She smiled at me and nodded, then kneeled down to pat Ralph again. He coated her with doggie kisses.

"That's the sweet boy. Oh my, you love that," she cooed, scratching Ralphie's ears. "Yes Ralph, you're so very handsome."

She turned to me again. "May I let him off his leash? Does he fetch?"

"Yes, absolutely!" I said, trying not to sound too surprised.

Beatrice picked up a stray tennis ball and threw it. Whoa.

"Oh, he's lovely," she grinned, as Ralph bounded after the ball. "Bring him over anytime Finn."

"Thanks. Wow Mrs. Bienenstock, that's quite the arm you've got there."

She smiled at the compliment. "It's the tennis. I try to play every day. It's such a wonderful pastime, don't you agree?"

I nodded. "Yes maam."

"I hear you're quite a good tennis player Finn.

I wish Charlie would play," she said as Ralphie brought the ball back, all slobbery.

Beatrice didn't seem to mind. She threw it again.

Ralph was loving The Beatrice!

Hmm, it's funny what you don't know about people sometimes. You can always be pleasantly surprised.

I still felt bad about Charlie, and I saw the chance to redeem myself.

I cleared my throat. "Uh, Mrs. Bienenstock?"

"Yes Finn?"

"Well, Charlie being my best friend and all, he told me about seeing Dr. Jones and the little weight problem," I rambled. "And I was doing some checking, and Dr. Jones has a lot of alternatives to…"

"Thanks mate, but I've got it."

Beatrice and I both turned around. Charlie was in the doorway.

"Mum, I wanted to talk to you about how I'm going to make some changes and get healthy," Charlie started.

"Of course darling," Beatrice answered, surprised. "I'm so pleased." She did sound proud of him. She glanced at me and smiled.

Beatrice gave Ralph a kiss on the head. "Adieu for now, Ralph." (I think Ralph even sat up straighter.)

Beatrice turned to Charlie. "Let's sit on the patio."

I put Ralph back on his leash and grinned despite myself. "See you tonight hermano!" I flashed

Charlie the thumbs up.

I was proud of the big lug too, but of course I had to keep my steely exterior. I waved and was off. As I let Ralphie pull me across the lawn towards home, I pumped my fist.

CHAPTER 22

I got home feeling great, but I felt like I had one more thing to do. When Ralph and I walked through the door, Dad was cooking. He had a beer on the counter and the radio on. He likes to cook. He says it relaxes him. And he's pretty good.

I'm getting into cooking some stuff too, and it's pretty cool. It gives you control of what you're eating, and it's kind of a mini-accomplishment to make yourself something that's actually edible.

"Hey Dad," I started.

The phone rang and I grabbed it. It was Tom. He was calling to see if I wanted to walk over to Charlie's together. I told him that that would be great, but I wanted some time to talk to Fiona first. I filled him in on the Fiona situation, and how she hadn't been eating, and Mom and Dad had to take her out of dance.

Dad looked at me, as if to say 'hey don't spill the family secrets'. But Tom's a good friend and he wouldn't say anything. Turns out, his mom and my mom had been talking. His big sister went to the same ballet school and had the same kookoo-for-Cocoa-Puffs teacher. Too much drama for me.

I was going to hang out with Fiona for a bit. He was going to head over in a while and pick me up. I hung up the phone.

"Where are Mom and Fiona?" I asked Dad.

Dad turned around, like I had surprised him. He was obviously super distracted.

"Hey Finn. Your mom's at the grocery store and Fiona's in the den." He looked bummed as he said this, as if being in the den was the equivalent to falling off a cliff.

I grabbed some cheese and crackers and a few grapes. "I'm just going to go hang out with her," I said, starting out of the kitchen.

"Finn," Dad called me back. "Just don't tease her or anything. She's pretty upset. Your mom and I had to take her out of ballet."

He stopped. "Hold it, you just told Tom that," he backtracked. "How did you know?"

Crap. I forgot I didn't 'officially' know that.

"I just knew Dad," I said, to his surprised expression. I gave him my 'I'm a sensitive big brother' look and nodded.

I wasn't going to explain the glass-against-the-wall listening device, so I continued out of the room. He was so distracted that I knew he wouldn't interrogate me.

The funny thing about my sister and me, is that while we can fight like cats and dogs over stuff like the t.v. remote or the computer. Or a hat for that matter, we usually get along pretty well. She can be pretty fun when she's not being all prissy, like she has been every day lately.

When I got to the den, Fiona was slumped in my favorite chair (forgiven this time), t.v. on, flipping through a magazine that she seemed to be completely uninterested in. I could tell she wasn't interested in the t.v. program, because it was pro wrestling, and I didn't think she'd switch affiliations that quickly.

"Hey," I led.

"Hey," she answered back, all blah.

"What're you doing?" I tried.

"Nothing," she responded flatly.

"I pointed to the television. "Learning some new moves?" I joked.

My joke flew over her head and landed with a thud.

"No," she said, in a major bummed out tone.

Hmm. This wasn't going to be easy.

"Switch it if you want," she added. "I'm not really watching anything." She tossed the remote to me and attempted a small smile. Her eyes were red like she had been crying.

Oh man, I was starting to feel really bad for her.

Well, this was getting nowhere. Time for the direct approach.

"Fi, I'm really sorry about ballet," I attempted. "But it is pretty crazy for a teacher to tell you not to eat. And you do look kind of sick these days. And how are we supposed to wrestle if you've got all those bones sticking out?" I grinned. "I'll kick your butt. Not that I don't now."

No reaction.

I paused, then went for it. "Maybe if you just eat more."

"I can't go back to the ballet school," she sighed.

"What about another one?" I was pretty sure there were a couple of good dance schools in town. Not that I know about that stuff. "Or do tennis or,"

"Finn, can we just not talk about it," she cut in. Her eyes were all watery now. She sniffled.

Oh beautiful, I was making her cry again. I can't deal with tears.

"Anyway, I'm really sorry. And if you need anything, you know," I kind of trailed off. "I'm here."

Then I did the best thing I could do: distraction. I flicked the channel to this show we both like. We don't watch that much tube around here, but this show always makes you laugh.

And I hung out with my sister, not sure what else I could do to make her feel better.

About a half an hour later, the doorbell rang. Ralph barked, Dad called, "got it" and in walked the answer.

Tom appeared in the doorway to the den. "Hey Finn," he said, pumped. "Hey Fiona!"

I motioned him in. "Hey, grab a seat."

Fiona gave a quick smile and wave. I think she was still a little teary because she excused herself, which is very rare when Tom is here. She started to get up, averting her eyes.

Tom sat down. He looked at the magazine she was holding, and pointed to a skinny model. "Oh man, that's gross."

That caught Fiona's interest. "What?" She glanced over.

"Those girls look like sickly skeletons. I'd never go out with someone like that," he assured us.

"Why Tom?" I joked, "You've got them lined up at your house wanting you to take them to The Yogurt Pump?"

Tom laughed. "No but seriously, I like girls who can go out and eat and do stuff," he said. "Real girls."

Fiona looked at him and reached for a cracker and a piece of cheese. I had to physically restrain myself from rolling my eyes. However, Tom's magic was working.

"Yeah, my big sister was losing all this weight and my mom was freaking out," Tom continued.

He turned to Fiona. "She had some crazy dance teacher who told her not to have milk or yogurt," he laughed. "For no reason!"

Man, Tom is brilliant sometimes.

"Yeah, she was my ballet teacher too," Fiona admitted. "Come to think of it, she was pretty restrictive."

"So now my sister's going to this new place," he continued. "Some ballet dancer from New York moved here and started it."

Now Fiona was not only drooling over Tom, she was actually interested in what he was saying. "Really? Where?" She sat down again.

"It's over by the old market, Fi. They renovated one of the historic old market buildings," he told her. "Your mom called my mom about it a little while ago."

I don't know if it was how he used her nick-name or the thought of a new ballet class, but Fiona smiled for the first time in a while.

"Anyway," Tom finished, "She just started and she loves it. You should try it out. You're a good dancer too aren't you?"

Fiona blushed and shrugged. I made a mental note to tell Tom that he rocks.

CHAPTER 23

The sleepover that night was a blast. Charlie looked recharged, Tom was hilarious, and Xavier broke his record slices of pizza eaten at a sleepover. (But trust me, he burned it off playing table tennis.)

At one point, we were goofing around in the indoor pool. We were diving for coins, and Charlie was floating on this massive air mattress.

I thought to myself, 'Here we go again. We're jumping around like a bunch of maniacs and Charlie's laying down again.'

But then he surprised me.

"Cannonball contest!" he yelled out. Soon we were all jumping off the diving board, seeing who could make the biggest splash.

Even though we're all really good swimmers, (I'm ready to go for my lifeguard levels,) Josie was sitting on deck watching us.

I wasn't sure if she wanted to join us or strangle us. But she was being a sport, and we managed not to soak her in our shenanigans.

Later on, as we were watching a movie, all cozy in our sleeping bags in the pool house 'guest area', Charlie whacked me.

I looked at him.

"Thanks," he said.

"No problem," I chipped back. And we went back to the movie. That was us. Simple. To the point. No gushing here.

CHAPTER 24

Right. No gushing! Until a couple of days later when Charlie called me.

"Thank you thank you thank you! I love you mate! I owe you big-time!" Charlie nearly shouted into the phone.

"What?" I sputtered.

"Just met personal trainer," Charlie said breathlessly. "Here now! Must get back!"

I heard they had called the German trainer. I was surprised Charlie was so pumped up. And very curious!

I was over at his house in a snap. Josie met me at the door. I half-asked/half-yelled, "Hey Josie, how are you!" as I sprinted past her to the gym.

I flew to their gym doorway, then slowed down, getting back into my cool mode. I didn't want to look like a dweeb in front of the super pumped German dude.

"Hey Charlie," I said casually, flipping my chin toward him.

You know when you see people turn around

in slow motion, in movies and commercials and stuff? It was like that: Charlie turned around, the biggest smile I'd ever seen plastered across his face. As he stepped to the side, I saw her. Ga ga!

The German dude was a German dudette.

She turned and smiled at me, her ponytail swishing. She looked like a movie star – with muscles.

"Finn, meet Heidi, my new personal trainer," beamed Charlie, punching every word, as if he couldn't believe his luck.

"Hello Finn," she said brightly, with a cool accent. "Charlie and I are just getting to know each other."

My gaze shifted to Charlie who was nodding and grinning like an imbecile.

"I hear you helped Charlie get on the right track," Heidi added.

Now it was my turn to nod and grin like a blockhead.

"Your parents are Kate and John, right?"

Who?

Right. I snapped out of it.

"Yeah," I breathed. Well, sort of snapped out of it.

"They are really well liked in the fitness community," she continued.

I stood there, nodding like a zombie.

"Finn, it is so nice to meet you," she said, smiling. Then to Charlie, "Well buddy, we'd better get started."

Buddy?! I'm the only one who calls him that. Charlie gazed adoringly at Heidi. Okay, obviously he didn't mind.

I excused myself and exited. Charlie looked over and I mouthed "call me" while holding my pretend phone to my ear. He nodded.

I started backing out while staring at Heidi, and tripped backwards out of the gym. (Why do I keep doing this lately?)

"Are you okay Finn?" she asked, starting to come toward me.

No, no, I'm not okay, I thought. Save me Heidi.

"Yeah I'm good," I actually said.

Oh well. Charlie was on his way to being fit and healthy. In fact, he looked a little thinner already. No wait, that was just him, sucking in his gut.

THE NOTEBOOK

So here's some of the info I came up with, while I was investigating Charlie's situation.

It would make a great health project in school. But really, I had fun learning about healthy weight ranges because (to use a tennis term), it puts the ball in my court.

Did you notice I said 'healthy weight **ranges**? Yeah. We all come in different shapes and sizes.

I had a few other lightbulb moments...

Skinny doesn't mean fit. Charlie won't necessarily ever be skinny, and that's good for him. He's a big bear of a guy. But he is getting fit and active. (By the way, Fiona learned that too, and now she's back to her usual semi-fun self.)

The other thing I learned is, (and this is big): It's not that tough.

Just do something active, everyday. (Or

at least, most days.)

Charlie walks more (after Beatrice took away limo cruising as an activity) and generally moves more during the day.

AND he feels better. (He also feels better because he took control of his own habits.)

(Am I using brackets too much??)

Little things you do every day can really help!

SO WHAT'S THE DEAL WITH BMI?

Okay, so now you know this cool new term to impress your friends:

B.M.I., or body mass index.

We were actually going to call the book 'Be My B.M.I.' (Isn't that catchy?)

But then we got thinking that 'Balance It Out' is way better.

Keeping healthy IS all about balance. It's balancing what you're eating with activity. It's also balancing any bad habits (if you have them) with good ones.

So the more we thought about it, the more we liked it.

BMI is just one tool for checking healthy weight, and it's really a guide. Like, when we checked Xavier's BMI with Dad, he was 'underweight'. But he's the king of nutrition and Mr. Activity, and he feels great, so it was no big deal.

A really good thing is to go by how you

feel:

Do you have energy?

Do you feel good?

Are you active and eating healthy stuff every day?

When you finish a meal or snack, are you pleasantly satisfied, or uncomfortably stuffed? (You want the first one!)

With adults, they say that you can tell if you're in healthy weight zones by how your clothes fit. (If, all of a sudden, they become way too tight or too loose.) But since we're growing at different rates, we can't really do that.

I grew a couple of quick inches in height last year, and my pants got so short, I looked like I was expecting a flood!

If you're a preteen (or tween... love calling Fiona that), and you're getting ready for a growth spurt, it can be pretty easy to gain a couple of pounds. But those fluctuations (ups and downs) are just part of the whole growing process.

If you really have some concerns about your weight, talk to someone you trust: a parent, teacher, doctor, coach, older sibling, or whoever you feel comfortable chatting with. It's really no drama.

(Like Fiona should have talked to the folks instead of losing all that weight. And if you're wondering: nope I don't know what her BMI was. She wouldn't let me weigh her. I think she was embarrassed. Too bad,

because I would have been my usual com-
passionate self!)

COOL FACTS

Did you know:

*Calories are these little nuggets of energy that we take in (in food) and burn off as fuel? (If you look at any label, it will tell you how many calories are in a serving.)

*That muscle weighs more than fat? (This is good to know, because sometimes, when we start exercising and eating better, we might not notice a big difference on the scale right away. If you're losing fat but building up some muscle, you might not see big changes in numbers, but you'll feel better!)

*That your brain takes about 30 minutes to realize you're full? (So don't chow down too fast, and give your brain time to catch up. If you want seconds, just wait a few minutes and see if you're still hungry.)

*Why they call some food 'empty calories'? It's because there's little or no nutritional value (stuff like vitamins, calcium, iron, protein, etc.) for the calories. Take soda for example. (In Canada we call it 'pop'.) I love it, but I really limit it to about once a week. Sometimes I have juice and add a little soda water. It's not too sweet, and it has a little fizz. So when you have a snack, eat something that's going to give you flavor AND do you a favor. (Hey, I'm a poet and I didn't know it!)

*The more muscle mass you have, the higher your metabolism? So, even by just sitting around, you burn more calories if your muscles are fit and strong.

*The safe rate of weight loss is 1 to 2 pounds a week? It's the same for weight gain. That's why lifestyle modification is so important if you want to make changes. Our bodies don't work well with drastic changes. (Don't they say patience is a virtue?)

*That fat is a major fuel for us? We use fats for energy when we do stuff like walking, swimming, riding bikes, running, and other aerobic exercise. So we need some fat. But just like a car doesn't need to carry around an extra gas tank, we don't need to carry a lot of excess fat either.

*That chocolate milk is an awesome post-exercise drink? (That's win-win.

*Different activities burn different numbers of calories. Higher intensity sports like running, dancing (I know Fiona – not a sport!), soccer, a good hard game of tennis, cross country skiing (which we do in Canada in winter), and hoops are just a few examples of activities that burn a high number of calories. Raking leaves, taking your dog for a walk, and going for a nice easy bike ride are good calorie burners too. Some of the activities that don't burn as many calories are the ones you can do for longer, so it all evens out. It's all about being active (a little or a lot) every day.

SMALL THINGS WE CAN DO EVERY DAY

Some of you may already be super in-volved in sports. Maybe you compete or play on a team or two.

Some of you may have your favor-ite activities already, and have a pretty healthy lifestyle.

And some of you might want to start getting a little healthier.

Whichever road you're coming from, I think these are pretty good reminders for all of us:

*Eat breakfast! Even if you don't have a lot of time, have something like a smoothie, fruit, a muffin, some cheese, or whatever's easy. Eating breakfast kick starts your engine, getting your metabolism turned up. While I'm at it, don't skip any meals. It just slows down your engine.

*Walk or ride your bike when you have to get somewhere, and it's safe to do it.

*Have some healthy, portable snacks with you when you're at school or out. That way, you won't get too hungry and go crazy eating junk later.

*Get your butt out of your chair when you can. When I do homework, if I'm stuck on something, I get up and stretch, walk around, or take Ralphie for a walk instead of staring blankly at the computer screen. You'll think better too, so you'll get your homework done faster! When I'm watching t.v., I get up every once in a while also, so I don't have a permanent imprint on the couch. You don't have to do jumping jacks. You can grab a sip of water. Just get your backside off the sofa.

*Did you know that, if you're watching t.v., you burn more calories while sitting up than if you're laying down? (Plus, you can see the screen the right way!) Sometimes I like to flake out on the couch too, but usually I try to stay upright. It's a little habit that helps

*Drink water! Have a water bottle with you at school or wherever you're hanging

out. (And don't just drink sweet drinks when you're thirsty. You'd be surprised at how many extra calories and sugar sneak into you!)

*Get out and play! Yeah yeah, I know that we're not little kids anymore. But everyone likes to play. (Case in point: Last year, we were training with skipping ropes, and Davis did double dutch! He was awesome! I, on the other hand, got tangled up. But it was fun.) Have you got a skipping rope? How about a basketball hoop in your neighborhood? If you have a group of kids, you can play all kinds of hide and seek type games (as long as everyone plays safe, sets boundaries, and watches out for each other). Have you ever played 'virus', where everyone hides and whenever someone gets caught, they join the kid who's 'it'. So after a while, you've got a bunch of you looking for one or two kids. It's fun. (I'll have more ideas on my website.)

*Be aware of how much time you spend in front of the t.v., computer, on your phone, iPad, or whatever. Add it up. You might be surprised. One time, I was on my screen for two hours. I don't know where the time went, and I felt kind of crappy afterward. I had missed the best part of an afternoon. Plus Ralph was miffed. A lot of kids I know have a limit. I've got to tell you, since I started keeping track of my screen time and keeping it at a decent limit, Mom and Dad have backed off timing me on it.

*Shut off all your screens a while before you go to bed, so your brain can get ready for bed too. We're not allowed to be on screens or computers within an hour of hitting the hay. (Supposedly it makes it harder to go to sleep. And good sleep is linked to healthy weight. I can see that. When I'm tired, I'm always reaching for extra munchies to perk up.)

*Don't just shove food in your mouth because you're bored. Or bummed out. Or stressed. Seriously, have something else in mind to do instead. I take Ralph for a walk. Xavier shoots hoops. Tom hits a tennis ball against a backboard. Chris dances or kicks around her soccer ball. Sometimes she borrows Ralph and takes him for fetch. (He's happy to help!) And now Charlie belts out a few tunes.

*When we have snacks, we're not allowed to eat right out of the bag or box. (Conversely, I once saw Charlie snarf down a whole bag of zesty nacho chips. At the end, after he burped, he couldn't believe he'd eaten the whole thing!) Put stuff in a bowl or plate. That way, you know how much you're having.

*When you're hanging out with your friends, don't just sit around someone's family room all the time. Plan some active stuff. Maybe a hike, or meeting up for a swim. Or, under the 'this is way more fun than I thought it would be' category: bowling!

*Put on music when you're doing chores, cleaning up your room, whatever. You can't help but move a little more when there's a good beat.

Then there's N.E.A.T....

N.E.A.T.

Dr. James Levine, a researcher at the Mayo Clinic (this big, world-famous hospital in Minnesota, U.S.A.) coined the term 'N.E.A.T.' for people who move all the time - fidget, get up to get stuff often, tap their fingers, whatever.

N.E.A.T. stands for 'Non-Exercise Activity Thermogenesis'. (Try saying that ten times fast!) Thermogenesis just means 'making heat'. (I looked it up.) Remember, our bodies produce heat when we burn calories.

Dr. Levine and his team found that people who move more throughout the day tend to keep weight off more than people who don't. They're always moving, so it keeps their metabolism running a little faster. So they burn more calories. As Charlie would say, that's brilliant!

The poster boy for NEAT is someone

like Xavier. Seriously, he is always in motion!

UNHEALTHY CHOICES AND HEALTHY ALTERNATIVES:

Remember when we had brownies and some junk food for our movie night? Like I say, I love the stuff... in smaller doses.

But I've got to tell you, the more I eat healthy foods, the more I appreciate them too. So we go for the healthier foods and snacks first. We eased into eating healthier foods most of the time, so I didn't feel like I was cut off my old favorites. (I know some people who don't eat any junk food, and they don't miss it.)

There are some types of fast food that I just don't like anymore. After eating at one place, my stomach felt like it had a boulder in it!

Anyway, here's my little list of some better snacks:

If you feel like something salty: Try pretzels, cheese and crackers, or some of the baked snack chips or rice crackers they have out now. (Just watch it so you don't eat too much salt. Lots of salt is crappy for you too.) Also, I love pistachios, and the fact that you have to shell them means you'll pace yourself. Air popped popcorn is also awesome!

If you feel like something sweet: Have some fruit, make yourself a smoothie, or have just a little dark chocolate. (It's pretty satisfying if you need a chocolate fix.) If you want a frozen treat, try the ones made with real fruit as opposed to the ones with just sugar, color, and water.

If you feel like something rich (those foods that usually have a lot of fat): Try low fat yogurt, frozen yogurt (Greek yogurt is awesome), or sherbet.

So, these are just a few ideas. There are tons of good options out there!

THE CELERY THING

Remember when Chris said that you wouldn't gain any weight eating celery, because you'd burn up the few calories by chewing and digesting?

Do you know how many calories are in a stalk of celery? Depending on the size, around 5 calories! So it's true!

Saying that, lots of people add something to make celery a little more interesting, like a healthy dip, or hummus.

I wonder how many of us had the old 'ants on a log' when we were small: celery with peanut butter and a few raisins on top.

The celery thing made me curious.

I looked up some **grab and go** snack foods that pack an energy punch, and are either low in calories, or have super healthy calories. Check it out in my next section!

SUPER HEALTHY SNACKS:

So trust me, I l-o-v-e junk food as much as you do. But like I said, in my house, moderation is the key.

The other key is making healthy snacks and meals really accessible. So when I get home after school or tennis, the healthy stuff is right there, ready to eat.

So if you have this kind of stuff around (check out my list, below), try to eat it first, then you won't feel so bad if you indulge (a little) in the junky stuff:

*Cheese and crackers. The softer the cheese, the better it is for you. Or get lower fat varieties.

*Nacho chips and salsa. Try the baked kind.

*Trail mix. You can buy it pre-made or

better yet, make your own. We call it GORP (Good Old Raisins and Peanuts). Mom used to make up a big bag for canoe trips when she was a teenager, back in the olden days. (Sorry Mom!) And you don't just use raisins and peanuts... almonds, dried cranberries or other fruit, carob or chocolate chips, coconut, sunflower seeds... the list goes on!)

*Veggies and hummus. (You can get the easy baby carrots.)

*Dried apricots.

*Almonds. (We always have a bowl of slow roasted almonds so we can just grab a handful whenever we want.)

*Yogurt. The Greek stuff has lots of protein.

*Bagel and almond butter or peanut butter.

*Fig newtons. (The figs are surprisingly nutritious and they're easy to take with you.) You can also get apple or other kinds of newtons.

*Bowl of cereal or oatmeal. (You can get packets and microwave it with milk if you're in a rush.)

*Yes, the classic: fruit. (I'm an apple guy myself.)

*Smoothie. This is my go-to snack. If you have some fruit, yogurt, milk, or a little juice (with water), you can make an awesome smoothie in seconds! The quickest smoothie ever is chocolate milk and a banana. (I add some white milk too so it's not too sweet.)

*Milk or chocolate milk. Wholesome with a capital W! (And delish with a capital D.) We get low fat milk. Some of my friends drink almond or soy milk too.

*I love baked stuff, so if you can make or have lower fat muffins or whatever, awesome. (Mom substitutes healthier ingredients a lot of the time when she bakes, like applesauce for some of the butter.)

Talk to whoever's buying the groceries in your house. Go along if you can sometimes, and help pick out some healthy snacks.

FOOD AND MOOD

I've got to tell you something. When I'm pumped up and excited about something, I tend to want to eat. When I'm stressed, I have no appetite.

For most people, it's the opposite. You want to see Xavier pile through food when he's stressed – it's not a pretty sight!

Remember when I wrote down that cookies were a big mood booster for Charlie? Yeah, well, he's learned to do other things and not depend on food to make him feel better.

One thing he didn't realize is that exercise is a mood booster too. Yep, so stuff like going for a walk or hike, a bike ride, shooting some hoops, or whatever, can make you feel better!

So now Charlie might have a cookie. But he depends more on activity to make him feel better. Like creaming his best friend in table tennis. (Who knew?) Or playing

Frisbee, or something like that. And then there's the singing. (Luckily he's a good singer.)

What makes you feel good?

DON'T BE A YOYO

Hey, have you ever heard of yoyo diets?

It's when someone goes on a diet and loses some weight.

Then they get sick of it, start eating all kinds of junk again and gain back a whole bunch of weight.

Then they feel crappy, so they go on another diet, and lose weight.

But then they fall off the wagon again and start eating too much crappy stuff. And they gain a few more pounds.

So... up, down, up, down, just like a yoyo.

You get my point.

People do that with exercise too sometimes: They get really active and fit, but then they aren't really having fun, or get really busy with other stuff, and then they stop exercising. Completely.

But then they feel crappy, so they go back to the gym or pool or track or whatever. They try to exercise a lot to make up for what they missed. But then they're really not having fun and they stop.

It's not great to be like a yoyo when it comes to eating or exercise. Health and fitness experts say you should work good habits into your **lifestyle**.

That means trying to be active and eat healthy foods day to day, and not kicking yourself in the butt if you have a few blips in your new healthy lifestyle. So if you have a lazy day or two, don't get frustrated and stop. Just get back at it with a positive attitude!

And pick physical activities that you like! Everyone's different and there are tons of different things you can do to keep fit.

Trust me, I know.

But that's our next adventure!

MY EMBARRASSING, HUMBLING STORY ON JUDGING PEOPLE.

(Can't believe I'm telling you this.)

Remember when I told Charlie that no one was judging him? That was a spur of the moment reply, but it's the truth.

I learned it the hard way.

A couple of years ago, Mom and I were driving to pick up a couple of movies one day, and, in between fiddling with the radio, I saw this guy out walking. He was a pretty big guy.

This is bad, but as we passed him I said, "Look at that fat guy." (Yes, I was young and immature.)

Mom looked at me and started in. "Don't you judge people. That guy is out walking and trying to keep fit while you're sitting on your butt in this car. You should have a lot of respect for that guy. Do you even know anything about that guy?"

My response: "Uh."

So then she pulled the car over and said, "Come on."

Oh crap.

The guy was walking toward us. Mom called out, "Hey Richard!"

The guy smiled as he approached. "Hi Kate, how are you?"

"I'm great thanks," Mom replied warmly. "Richard, this is my son Finn," she said as he reached out to shake my hand.

"Nice to meet you Finn!" he said sincerely.

(Yes, I felt like a worm.)

"Tell me," continued Mom, "Are you still at the same dojo?"

"Sure am," he nodded. "Drop by sometime."

"We will," said Mom. "Nice to see you."

So it turned out this guy was, like, a second-degree black belt, because we did drop by the dojo (the place where they practice karate,) a few days later. And Richard was pretty amazing.

I learned a huge lesson. So now, when I see someone out walking or being active, I think that's awesome. They're making an effort and that's a big deal.

If you have a friend, classmate, or family member who's struggling with his or her weight one way or the other, do me a favor: Don't tease, bully, or look down on them.

Support and encourage them!

A comment that you might think is funny might stick with someone else long after you've forgotten.

I've really learned to be a good example and be a good friend.

Remember, we all come in different shapes and sizes and that's awesome. It's all about being active and healthy and feeling good!

(So be good to yourself too.)

Drop in and see me at my website! I'm at:
www.fitfiles.net

Sue and I will have some more info, links, recipes, activity and game ideas, and a spot for questions.

Lots of cool stuff you can check out.

ACKNOWLEDGMENTS
AND THANKS

Sue and I couldn't have done this by ourselves.

We'd like to thank a few people who are bigtime experts in their field: Jacklynn Humphrey PDt, RD, a registered dietitian and Wellness Facilitator at Capital Health, in Halifax, Nova Scotia. When it comes to good, healthy food, she's a peach!

Dr. Sara Kirk, who's the Canada Research Chair in Health Services Research at Dalhousie University, and the Director of Applied Research Collaborations for Health. We could go on, but let's just say she knows what she's talking about when it comes to healthy weight and activity!

Dr. Laurene Rehman, a professor and researcher in Leisure Studies at Dalhousie University's School of Health and Human Performance. One of the things she studies is recreation and leisure time in kids and youth and how they affect our health.

How cool is that?

Their feedback was appreciated and invaluable. Any inaccuracies in the book are Sue's fault, not theirs. (Sue told me to say that.)

We also want to thank Dawson Tilley (no relation, but obviously a good guy with a name like that) for reading the very first draft of the book. Neve MacCormack was our British connection, reading the manuscript and making sure we didn't mess up on anything from the U.K. (Needless to say, Charlie was happy about that.) Ethan and Kiel Rehman, a couple of great guys who can hang out with my gang anytime. Peggy Lugar, a former P.E. teacher, and one of the most awesome teachers we know. Derek Estabrook, marketing whiz (and really fast runner). Tom Stender, who let Sue know when she was getting too retro. Carolina Stender, thanks for the great line.

Sue wanted to mention two professors who really inspired her to pursue fitness and health: Dr. Phil Campagna from Dalhousie University, and Dr. Bob McMurray from The University of North Carolina – Chapel Hill. (There's nothing like a great teacher.)

Sue also wants to thank her friends and family for being supportive and putting up with her while we finished this. (Again, her words!)

Mark, Tom, Carolina, and of course, Skyler... you're the best!

LET ME TELL YOU ABOUT SUE COMEAU!

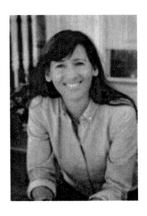

Sue has been interested in fitness and health ever since the days when she used to volunteer with kids at the local YMCA. She has coached, taught and worked with kids and young adults ever since.

Sue's a Certified Exercise Physiologist. She has a B.Sc. in Kinesiology (that's human movement studies) from Dalhousie University. Sue also has a Masters in Exercise Physiology from The University of North Carolina – Chapel Hill.

A funny thing happened while Sue was doing her Masters… She discovered she loved to write. She writes books, screenplays, and health and fitness articles.

She lives in Halifax, Nova Scotia with her husband, two kids, and their Labrador retriever (kid #3).

When she's not playing with her kids (her favorite pastime), she loves to run and play tennis (yes)!

Come see us at my website
www.fitfiles.net and learn more!